# HE RESTORED MY SOUL

## In the Valley of the Shadow of Cancer

**Charlaine F. Price**

**Limits of Liability and Disclaimer of Warranty**

The author and publisher shall not be liable for your misuse of this material. This book is strictly for informational and educational purposes. The use of short quotations or occasional page copying descriptive of personal encounters is permitted. Unless otherwise indicated, Scriptures are taken from the New International Version Bible. Some Bible versed have been paraphrased.

**Warning – Disclaimer**

The purpose of this book is to educate, encourage and empower. The author and/or publisher do not guarantee that anyone following these techniques, suggestions, tips, ideas, or strategies will overcome chronic illness. The author and/or publisher shall have neither liability nor responsibility to anyone with respect to any loss or damage caused, or alleged to be caused, directly or indirectly by the information contained in this book.

ISBN 978-1-941749-72-2
Library of Congress Number 2017912715
Cover Design: MS Design & Photography
Photographer: Michael Simmons
Editor: Deborah Levine Enterprises, LLC
Interior design: Laura Brown

4-P Publishing, Chattanooga, TN 37411

Rolling down the hall of the dimly lighted hallway to the emergency room, you could hear me crying out to God because Psalm 23 could not comfort me, for my focus was on fear, not God. He was not comforting me in the valley of the shadow of cancer.

"HELP ME!"

"Help me, LORD! You promised, you promised me, and I'm standing on your promises. I need you right now, right now! I feel so all alone. Where are you, God? Where are you!!! Didn't you tell me to go ahead and take that Chemo? Answer me!"

# About the Author

Charlaine F. Price is a Speaker, Teacher, Entrepreneur, and Licensed Professional Counselor (LPC). She is the wife of John L. Price, and they have four adult children, Corery Price, Corecia Harbour, and stepsons Donnell and Kerry Price. They have six delightful and intellectual grandchildren.

Charlaine retired as educator and administrator from the Hamilton County Schools after thirty-three years of service. She was the recipient of several awards during her tenure with the school system. She was honored at Riverside High School as Teacher of the Year (1978), at Tyner High School as Counselor of the Year (1988), and the Tennessee Vocational Administrator of the Year for the state of Tennessee (2000).

Charlaine has served as President of many professional organizations and served on the Board of several local organizations. She is the former Director of Christian Education and Youth Sunday School Teacher at Greater Tucker Missionary Baptist Church. She assisted the pastor with Pre-Marital Counseling and coordinated the Couples Ministry for more than ten years.

Her community service includes volunteering to assist the chaplains with the Well-Spring Program at Memorial Hospital and serving on the Children of Abuse Review Team (CART) for the Tennessee State Department of Human Services.

Charlaine is a trained Stephen Minister, a Licensed Professional Counselor (LPC), a Certified Christian Counselor, and a member of the American Association of Christian Counselors (AACC). She obtained degrees from Tennessee State University, the University of Tennessee at both Chattanooga and Knoxville, and from the Psychological Studies Institute (PSI)/Richmont University. She has several specialized degrees and certifications, but she is proudest of her B.A. "Born Again" Christian degree.

Charlaine is a Christian Therapist with more than twenty-seven years of experience. She is the founder of the Preventive Christ-Centered Options (PCO) Counseling Service and has helped adolescents, individuals, couples, families, and business organizations make successful transitions. Her logo tagline, "Serving People God's Way," is named for her certificate program in Biblical Counseling from the American Association of Christian Counseling.

PCO Counseling Service
Heritage V Building
5916 Brainerd Road, Suite 110
Chattanooga, TN 37411
www.pcocounseling.com

# Dedication

This book is dedicated to my family, and particularly to my daughter, Corecia. While I live in Chattanooga, my daughter lives a two-hour drive away in Nashville, Tennessee. She insisted I take my cancer treatments in Nashville at Vanderbilt University so that she could help care for me while my son, Corery, and her Dad, my husband John, were working. God knew my future and positioned her as a stay-at-home mom.

I am so grateful to Corecia for inviting me into her home and providing me with around-the-clock care. Caring for two small children and me is no easy task, but you made it work. So many days I depended on your physical strength when I was unable to get out of bed on my own. I also depended on your knowledge of the immune system to help me understand the medical jargon in the doctor's office at the beginning of my treatment.

To my wonderful son-in-law, Janaar: thank you for getting me to my cancer treatments when I had to be in Nashville before daylight during the winter months for those 7:00 a.m. lab appointments. You are an expert at maneuvering through traffic. I was never late for an appointment.

# Acknowledgements

I acknowledge with gratitude and love my village of caregivers and supporters:

My devoted husband, John, who drives me back and forth to Nashville for my cancer treatments at Vanderbilt. Thank you for being there during my infusions reminding me that God is looking after me and that he will never leave me or forsake me. Your faith in God has truly carried me through this cancer journey.

My compassionate son, Corery, for his sacrifice by moving in-house to care for me during the hours his Dad worked. His move provided me with around-the-clock care.

My brother, Thomas Finley, Sr., shared his nurse practitioner skills with his baby sister.

My precious grandchildren, Madison, Makenzie, and Xavier, who installed Marco Polo on my iPhone so they could entertain me with musical, magic tricks, laughter, and kisses.

My dedicated nephew, Troy Finley and his caring wife, Carla, made frequent visits from Atlanta to pray for God's strength to carry me through my valley days.

My concerned niece, Pamela Burrows in St. Louis

lifted my spirit with her inspirational texts and calls of encouragement.

My knowledgeable niece, Mona Finley, owner of Glenn Lakes Pharmacy in Sugarland, Texas, for her advice on alternative prescriptions for blood transfusion and a non-addicting prescription for pain.

My oncologist, Dr. Madan Jagasia, and Sheldon Lacy, his Assistant in the Hematology and Stem Cell Transplant Department at Vanderbilt Hospital and the Vanderbilt staff for treating "me the individual, and not just the disease."

My longtime friend and college roommate, attorney Earlyne McCallister Thomas in St. Louis continues to keep in touch. I wouldn't have gotten out of bed some mornings, but your inspiring quotes and memes helped me start another day's journey. I thank you for that and for continuing to keep me in your thoughts and prayers daily.

My friend Dr. Laura Royster in Detroit who gifted me with Louise Hay's book, *You Can Heal Your Life.*

My long-time girlfriend, Dr. Joyce Hardaway CEO of Hardaway Consulting Services for asking to accompany me on my doctor's visit. I will forever be grateful to you for asking to go with me to the oncologist and for being there with an extra set of ears to listen.

My friend Carolyn Jones, CEO of CJ Enterprise for the empowering card with the poem, *"What Cancer Cannot Do."*

My dedicated Prayer Warriors: Sis. DeVonne Fouche, Sabbath School Teacher; Elder Martin Lister, former Pastor of Orchard Park Seventh Day Adventist Church; Greater Friendship Primitive Baptist Church Members, Elder Reginald L. Yates, Pastor of Greater Friendship Primitive Baptist Church, and Members Alton Carson, Loretta Harris, and Barbara Scott of Greater Tucker Missionary Baptist Church, Rev. Gary Hathaway, Pastor of Greater Tucker Missionary Baptist Church.

My Teaching Leader, Susan Laramore and class members at the Bible Study Fellowship (BSF) program in Chattanooga, Tennessee for their support.

My former student, Robin (Dee) Sales, President and Founder of the Society of Bold Godly Wo-Men (BGW) who sponsored my first public testimony during the Annual American Breast Cancer Week at Chattanooga State Community College with the theme, "All Cancers Matter."

My former students, Beverly Bridges, Susan Freeman, Cedric Means, and the Riverside High School

Students for honoring me at their 40th Class Reunion with flowers, hugs, and memories.

My former Link Sisters: Dr. Joyce Hardaway, LaFonde McGee, and Ollie Reed for the home-cooked meals they provided my first week home from Nashville.

My past presidents and other Delta Sorors: Angel Ulmer for the beautiful throw that keeps me warm, Lucrecia Ramsey and Christine Hicks, and other members for the monetary gifts and get-well cards.

My former colleague, Barbara Whitehead, and the former students enrolled in Principles for a Spirit-filled Life Class at the Eastgate Senior Center. I am also grateful to Beverly Scott and the other women who made up our class. You all are an excellent support group.

My former Howard High School Class of '66 classmates: Wanda Stone for the four-leaf clover of healing, Rosetta Johnson, Rosetta Williams, Laurel Buttram, Henry Slayton, Charles Ballard, Linda Qualls, Patricia Sparks, Linda Dotson, Marian Higginbottham and others for your cards, calls, text messages, and loving kindness at our class meetings and morning walks. You guys mean the world to me.

My loving neighbors, Fartema Fagin and Debbie

Blansit for your caring deeds and support. My Facebook friends, Harold Bush and those who posted their prayers and support statements on my Facebook Page.

My inspiring S.W.A.T. Book Camp Coach, Laura Brown of 4-P Publishing. Thank you for sharing your "Book-Writing" skills, creative formatting gift and community networks.

My Book Editor, Ms. Deborah Levine of The Writers' Guru for helping me organize and tell my story.

Michael Simmons of MS Design & Photography for capturing my story on the cover of this book.

The Holy Spirit – Thank you for being my compass for this journey (Proverbs 3:5-6).

# Foreword

It is an absolute honor to write the forward to *He Restored My Soul: In the Valley of the Shadow of Cancer,* an inspiring and passionate book about the testimony and experience of Charlaine Price. Each year, over a hundred thousand persons die from cancer, men, women, and children alike. The thought of cancer, or any other chronic disease, can be frightening, disheartening, frustrating, and hard to understand. Many times, the question *why* is asked, but often, there is no answer.

In this manuscript, Charlaine shares about risk factors, signs, symptoms, prevention and treatment of various types of cancer. As you read each chapter, be prepared to receive more than just book knowledge about the effects and manifestation of this chronic disease. Instead, you will gain a deeper understanding of the struggle, the trials and the perseverance of a God-fearing cancer survivor. You will also experience genuine encouragement, support, and biblical guidance while learning about God's health plan for your life.

Preventing and managing a chronic condition like cancer, may not be easy, but Charlaine's testimony of courage, determination, and complete trust in God gives hope to all individuals traveling through "The Valley of the Shadow of Cancer."

Chelauna Sterling, B.S., MPH
Chronic Disease Public Health Educator
Chattanooga-Hamilton County Health Department

# PREFACE

I cried out with tears rolling down my checks as they wheeled me into the Emergency Room, "God, God, Oh my God! I need you to help me! Help me please, help me! The attendants assumed that I was in pain, but I was dealing with fear, not pain. I was all alone, and I could not feel the Holy Spirit. I cried out again, "God, where are you?" "God, you promised me, and I am standing on your promise right now LORD. Right now, don't leave me!" God, didn't you tell me to take that chemo? You led me to scripture John 2:19, destroy this temple, and I will raise it in three days.

The doctors and interns could not help staring at my bloody red lips puffed with puss and inflammation. What they could not see was the red rash scattered across my back and breast. What mainly got their attention was my mouth. They were afraid I was either having a side effect to the medication or had developed a deadly viral infection called SJS, "Steven Johnson's Syndrome." The word spread throughout the ER that a patient was there with SJS. I cried out, "Oh My God!"

God and I spent five years of spiritual training to prepare for the Valley of the Shadow of Cancer. Multiple Myeloma (MM) is a blood plasma cancer that attacks the bones. God trained me as a prayer warrior and later anointed me with the Holy

Spirit to declare His works. He taught me lessons which are outlined in the book to prepare me for the trials of life. These lessons will serve as guidelines to help you prepare for your trials of life. He put people in my life, lead me to nutritional events, gave me healing scriptures, and taught me what I needed to do to receive his promises. I am sharing this knowledge with you as God's Plan for our health, nutrition, and wellness. The many scriptures cited in my story are from both the traditional King James Version of the Bible and the New International Version.

I accepted God as my Healer, and because of it, I have been in communion with God over the last five years, preparing and training to fight this enemy, CANCER. The training was necessary because there is no known cure for cancer and the diagnosis usually leads to a prognosis of two to five years to live. I had to accept the diagnosis or be in denial, but I did not accept the prognosis of 2-5 years to live.

My cancer journey is charted as smoldering up to Mount Metastasis and down the Valley of Side Effects in the ER to the disappointment station of a Set Back before the announcement of Remission that takes me to the Promise Land of Restoration.

On the journey, I learned about God's plan of

proper diet. Biblical food is suggested as our guide to nutrition, health, and wellness as outlined in the Bible as the prevention to chronic diseases and it has been said to cure many people with cancer. Only God knows how long I have on this earth or how long it will take for me to fulfill His purpose.

# A POEM OF MY PHILOSOPHY

Cancer is so limited...

It cannot cripple LOVE

It cannot shatter HOPE

It cannot corrode FAITH

It cannot eat away PEACE

It cannot destroy CONFIDENCE

It cannot kill FRIENDSHIP

It cannot shut out MEMORIES

It cannot silence COURAGE

It cannot reduce ETERNAL LIFE

It cannot quench the SPIRIT

Author Unknown

# CHAPTER 1:
# HELP ME, LORD!!!

*He Restoreth My Soul. He leadeth me in the paths of righteousness for His name's sake. Yea, though I walk through the valley of the shadow of death, I will fear no evil; for Thou art with me; Thy rod and Thy staff they comfort me.*

*(Psalm 23:3)*

We cannot have Faith in God if we do not trust Him. I thought I trusted God until I reached the emergency room feeling all alone. It is hard to breathe when life is not fair. My prayers are going up, and it feels like God is not there. Help me, LORD!!! After crying out to God, I refocused on seeking Him. He relieved my fear with the "Psalm of Comfort" once I put my focus on him and not my side effects.

You will experience and witness the devastation of cancer. I can certainly identify with the scripture in (Psalm 23:4) "Thou I walk through the Valley of the Shadow of Death, I will fear no evil for thou art with me." This scripture is the one to assure you and me that God will take us through our trials if we trust Him. You cannot have Faith without Trusting God.

Allow me to share with you that which happened to me on my journey with Cancer. I call it my Valley Journey because in my early diagnosis I wandered around for five years just being monitored. Those years were called my smoldering years which was part of my diagnosis. I discovered that God gave me this time to smolder in the valley to teach me the spiritual things I needed to know to survive this battle with cancer. I had to learn that this battle is not mine, it's the LORD's. I dreaded the need for chemo or radiation, but when miraculous cures did not come, and the cancer metastasized, I had to resort to medical treatment.

This is a remarkable true story about adversity, anger, and fear of physical brokenness during my battle with cancer. You will witness the physical destruction of the temple (my body) and how I lost my focus on God and started to worry about myself due to my controlling nature. You should note that when I took my focus off God and put it on Self, I felt all alone and fear overtook me. God is faithful, and you will see how God raised the temple in three days as he promised me when I fasted and prayed about the uncertainty of having to take chemo. Too often we are in "reactive mode" not thinking of Proverbs 3:5-6 which asks us to trust God.

I have incorporated a poem written by an unknown author, *"What Cancer Cannot Do."* It is a great attention getter when I do my public speaking events. I discovered this poem during my stay at the MEET Ministry, a Missionary Education & Evangelistic Training Program in Huntington, Tennessee where I paid for services to cleanse my body and teach me all about caring for myself the naturopathic way.

When I look back over the journey and see where God has brought me with Cancer, I can see

His favor, and I am truly grateful. While smoldering in the wilderness, God, the Holy Spirit taught me so much to prepare me for the Valley of the Shadow of Cancer. You will witness "The Shadow of Cancer" and how He directed me while smoldering through the Valley of brokenness, before taking me up the Mountain to Metastasis, down the Valley of Side Effects, only to discover Setbacks before restoring me to the Promised Land of Remission."

There are many scriptures relevant to my journey but, there are four scriptures that gave me hope and encouragement to make the journey as I realized how God kept his promises:

1. *"You will not die, but live, to declare the works of the LORD." (Psalm 118:17)*

2. *"Destroy this temple, and in three days I will raise it up." (John 2:19)*

3. *"Trust in God with all your heart and lean not to your own understanding but, in all your ways acknowledge God and He will direct your path." (Proverbs 3:5-6)*

4. *"He restoreth my soul: he leadeth me in the paths of righteousness for his name's sake. Yea, though I walk through the valley of the shadow of death, I will fear no evil; for thou*

*art with me; thy rod and thy staff they com-*
*fort me." (Psalm 23:3-4)*

Cancer is no match for God. This declaration is in keeping with God's request to "declare the works of the LORD. The Epilogue summarizes "What Cancer Did Not Do." God kept his promises to me, and I want to be obedient and meet His request to inform the people by "declaring His Works." Declaring His Works educates, encourages, and empowers others experiencing trials. His declaration provides the knowledge necessary to trust in the LORD for their health and healing.

*My people are destroyed for lack of*
*Knowledge. (Hosea 4:6)*

# CHAPTER 2:
# ALL CANCERS MATTER

*There are many Cancers, but Breast Cancer is widely celebrated.*

*Let's recognize the common cancers and their symptoms.*

Cancer is a genetic disease that is caused by changes in genes that control the way our cells function, especially how they grow and divide. Genetic changes that cause cancer can be inherited from our parents. They can also arise during a person's lifetime because of errors that occur as cells divide, or because of damage to DNA caused by exposure to certain environmental elements. Cancer is the uncontrolled growth of abnormal cells in the body. It is named for the organ or type of cell in which it starts growing.

All cancers matter because we are all targets of this horrible disease. The lives of children, women, and men are affected by cancers of all kinds. Breast cancer has gotten much attention because tumors in the breast are easily identified and can be detected by touch. According to the American Cancer Society, a lump or mass is the most common symptom and can be found with regular "self-checks" of the breast. Other breast changes such as thickening, swelling, distortion, tenderness, skin irritation, redness, scales, nipple abnormalities, and discharge are visible. If left untreated, they begin to exhibit pain. There are so many other cancers, but now you know why breast cancer has gotten so much attention and been well celebrated.

Have we considered the breast cancer in

men? The American Cancer Society wants us to know Breast Cancer is not limited to only women. It affects men as well as women. They encourage men to get breast exams and watch for these possible symptoms: a lump or swelling, which is usually (but not always) painless, skin dimpling or puckering, nipple retraction (turning inward), redness or scaling of the nipple or breast skin, and discharge from the nipple. Sometimes a breast cancer can spread to lymph nodes under the arm or around the collar bone and cause a lump or swelling, even before the original tumor in the breast tissue is large enough to be felt. These changes are not always caused by can-

> Cancer has no respect for persons... We are all vulnerable to this disease.

cer. For example, most breast lumps in men are caused by gynecomastia (a harmless enlargement of breast tissue). Still, if you notice any breast changes, you should see a health care professional as soon as possible.

Cancer has no respect for persons. We all belong to the human race, and it does not matter whether we are black or white, male or female, young or old. We are all vulnerable to this disease. If you do not have cancer, you know someone, a friend or loved one who has cancer. Cancer dominates our society.

Cancer can be experienced by any human being. My dentist and I share the same cancer diagnosis. I thank God for him serving as a cancer partner with me. We share our treatment stories during my dental cleanings. I also have the same kind of cancer as the well-known news commentator, Tom Brokaw, and the two things we have in common is our age and birthday. We are both over the age of fifty and were born in February on the same day. The cancer we share is a rare type which attacks individuals age fifty and older. It is a bone cancer called Multiple Myeloma.

Multiple Myeloma is not one of the commonly diagnosed cancers. It is a bone cancer and is a cousin to Leukemia and Lymphoma. Myeloma is when affected cells are not able to function properly. The bones do not provide adequate marrow, and the marrow does not supply pure blood to help fight against germs, viruses or disease because the immune system is weakened. This cancer is often referred to as MM, and it is the second most common form of blood cancer in the United States. It is a type of cancer that develops in the soft, spongy tissue at the center of your bones, called bone marrow. It causes cancer cells to accumulate, where they crowd out healthy blood cells and can prevent your immune system from working properly. It is considered a long-lasting disease.

There are more than one hundred types of cancer. For the sake of this declaration, we will focus on the common types and their symptoms. Types of cancer are usually named for the organs or tissue where the tumors form. For example, lung cancer starts in cells of the lung, and brain cancer begins in cells of the brain. When they metastasize to other organs, they continue to be named for the original organ affected.

## Categories of Cancers

(Defined by the Type of Cell Where They Begin)

## Carcinoma

Carcinomas are the most common type of cancer. They are formed by epithelial cells, which are the cells that cover the inside and outside surfaces of the body. Carcinomas that begin in different epithelial cell types have specific names:

- Adenocarcinoma forms in epithelial cells that produce fluids or mucus.

- Basal cell carcinoma begins in the lower basal (base) layer of the epidermis, which is the outer layer of skin.

- Squamous cell carcinoma forms in squamous

cells, which are epithelial cells that lie just beneath the outer surface of the skin. They can be in the linings of many organs, including the stomach, intestines, lungs, bladder, and kidneys. Transitional cell car-cinoma forms in a type of epithelial tissue called transitional epithelium or urothelium. It is found in the linings of the bladder, ureters, and part of the kidneys (renal pelvis).

## Sarcoma

Sarcomas form in bone and soft tissues, including muscle, fat, blood vessels, lymph vessels, and fibrous tissue including tendons and ligaments. The most common types of soft tissue sarcoma are leiomyosarcoma, Kaposi sarcoma, malignant fibrous histiocytoma, liposarcoma, and dermatofibrosarcoma protuberans. Osteosarcoma is the most common bone cancer.

## Leukemia

Cancers that begin in the blood-forming tissue of the bone marrow are called leukemias. These cancers do not form solid tumors. Instead, large numbers of abnormal white blood cells (leukemia cells and leukemic blast cells) build up in the blood and bone marrow, crowding out normal blood cells. The low level of healthy blood cells can make it harder for the body to get oxygen to its tissues, control bleeding, or fight infections.

There are four common categories of leukemia: acute or chronic, and depending on the type of blood cell where the cancer originates (lymphoblastic or myeloid).

## Lymphoma

Lymphoma is cancer that begins in the lymphocytes (T cells or B cells). These are disease-fighting white blood cells that are part of the immune system. Abnormal lymphocytes build up in lymph nodes and lymph vessels, as well as in other organs of the body.

There are two main types of lymphoma: Hodgkin lymphoma, also called Reed-Sternberg cells, that form from B cells. Non-Hodgkin's lymphoma is a large group of cancers that start in lymphocytes. They can grow quickly or slowly and can form from T cells or B cells.

## Melanoma

Melanoma begins in cells that become melanocytes, which are specialized cells that make melanin, the pigment that gives skin its color. Most melanomas form on the skin, but melanomas can also develop in other pigmented tissues, such as the eye.

## Brain and Spinal Cord Tumors

Brain and spinal cord tumors are named based on the type of cell in which they originated and where the tumor first formed in the central nervous system.

## Germ Cell Tumors

Germ cell tumors are a type of tumor that begins in the cells that give rise to sperm or eggs. These tumors can occur almost anywhere in the body and can be either benign or malignant.

## Neuroendocrine Tumors

Neuroendocrine tumors form in cells that release hormones into the blood in response to a signal from the nervous system.

## Carcinoid Tumors

Carcinoid tumors are a type of neuroendocrine tumor. They are slow growing tumors that are usually found in the gastrointestinal system, most often in the rectum and small intestine. They may spread to the liver and other sites in the body.

## Common Sites of Cancers

American Cancer Society's most recent facts and figures 2017 annual report lists the ten cancers estimated to be the most diagnosed in 2017.

(American Cancer Society's current facts and figures annual report published on WebMD)

**1. Breast Cancer** - Unsurprisingly, breast cancer is predicted to be the most commonly diagnosed cancer among women. Breast cancer is the
second-leading cause of cancer deaths among
women. While breast cancer in men is a small
percent of all cases of breast cancer, it does occur.

**2. Prostate Cancer** - Prostate cancer is the third-
leading cause of cancer death among men. Early
prostate cancer has no symptoms, so regular exams
are imperative. Once the disease has advanced, men
may experience weak or interrupted urine flow, frequent urination, difficulty stopping and starting
urine flow, blood in the urine, and pain or burning
during urination. Very advanced prostate cancer
may spread to bones, which can cause pain in the
hips, spine, ribs and other areas.

**3. Lung and Bronchus** - Lung cancer is the second most commonly diagnosed cancer in the
United States. It is the leading cause of cancer
death in both men and women. Symptoms do not
usually occur until the cancer is advanced. They include a persistent cough, sputum streaked with
blood, chest pain, voice change, worsening shortness of breath, as well as recurrent pneumonia or

bronchitis. Eighty percent of lung cancer deaths in the U.S. are caused by smoking.

**4. Colorectal** - Like lung and prostate cancer, colorectal cancer can be hard to detect in the early stages, which may account for its high mortality rate. Symptoms include rectal bleeding, blood in the stool, changes in bowel habits or shape, feeling that the bowel is not completely empty, cramping pain in the lower abdomen, and decreased appetite or weight loss.

**5. Uterine Corpus** - Abnormal bleeding is often an early sign of this type of cancer. Women should report any abnormal bleeding or spotting to their physicians, especially if they are postmenopausal.

**6. Bladder** - Blood in the urine is a common symptom of urinary bladder cancer. Other symptoms include increased urgency, more frequent urination, or pain and irritation during urination.

**7. Melanoma (skin cancer)** - Skin cancer is the most frequently diagnosed cancer in the United States. Warning signs of skin cancers include changes in the size, shape, or color of a mole or other skin lesion. Also, be alert to the appearance of a new growth on the skin or a sore that doesn't heal.

**8. Thyroid** - A lump in the neck is the most common symptom of thyroid cancer. Other symptoms include a tight or full feeling in the neck, difficulty breathing or swallowing, hoarseness, swollen lymph nodes and pain in the neck or throat that doesn't go away.

**9. Kidney/Renal** - Like colorectal cancer, kidney cancer usually doesn't have any symptoms in its early stages. As the tumor progresses, symptoms may include blood in the urine, pain or a lump in the lower back or abdomen, fatigue, weight loss, fever or swelling in the legs and ankles.

**10. Non-Hodgkin's Lymphoma** - Non-Hodgkin's lymphoma is swollen lymph nodes. Other symptoms include lumps under the skin, chest pain, shortness of breath, abdominal fullness and loss of appetite, itching, night sweats, fatigue, unexplained weight loss and intermittent fever. These are common symptoms that could be warning signs of cancer.

# CHAPTER 3:
# BODY LANGUAGE

*Our body speaks to us in terms of symptoms.*

D id you know that our body speaks to us in the language of symptoms? Symptoms such as heartburn and depression may indicate cancer.

Here are nine symptoms you must not dismiss. They could be symptoms of cancer.

1. **Change in bowel habits:** If your bowel habits have changed in timing, size, amount or any other way, it could be indicative of colon cancer.

2. **Change in bladder habits**: This symptom is likely dismissed by women because we are no stranger to urinary tract infections. But, if you experience blood in your urine, experience urgency or pain, it is a good idea to get to the doctor.

3. **Unexplained pain:** Of all the symptoms, this one the most general. Pain is an indication that something is wrong — it's a smart idea to make sure that "something" is not cancer.

4. **A lump:** A lump in the neck could indicate a head or neck cancer, or a lymphoma. Lumps in the breast could also be indicative of cancer — but they could be cysts, too. If you have a lump in your body, talk to a doctor. He or she may be able to rule out the lump being cancer, but it is a good idea to know for sure.

5. **A non-healing sore throat**: During cold and flu season, you may be tempted to write off that scratchy sore throat, but the report says not to. It could point to laryngeal cancer or throat cancer.

6. **Unexplained weight loss**: Shedding pounds may be welcome news, but if you're dropping weight without drastically changing your diet or exercise regimen, it's worth investigating. Losing weight doesn't mean you have cancer, but it can signal that something is wrong with your body.

7. **Difficulty swallowing:** It could be a sign of esophageal cancer, or it could be another type of infection. It is best to know what's going on with confirmation from a physician.

8. **Bleeding:** Blood in the urine can indicate kidney or bladder cancer. If you are bleeding after menopause or after sex, it might be a sign of gynecological cancer such as cervical cancer.

9. **Change in a mole's appearance**: Of the 7 percent of people in the study that experienced this symptom, about 47 percent contacted their doctors — while 53 percent did not. A mole or freckle that changes in appearance could indicate a type of cancer. It is easy for physicians to rule out things like melanoma — but better to have it

checked out, as many melanomas can be re-moved.

Listen to your body because what you feel might be symptoms of cancer, so be on the look-out if something does not feel right. Know that God can heal all cancers because all cancers matter to God. Isaiah 53:5 says, He was wounded for our transgressions, buried for our iniquities, the chastisement of peace was upon Him, and by his stripes, we are healed. Psalm 107 says Jesus bore my sickness and carried my pain. For God sent His Word and healed me.

> Listen to your body because what you feel might be symptoms of cancer, so be on the lookout if something does not feel right

Thousands of people die each day from cancer. If it scares you, it is understandable. Whether you are trying to avoid cancer or beat it, or if you already have it, there is one powerful antidote to the fear and to the disease itself -knowledge. *The people perish for lack of knowledge." (Hosea 4:6)* Knowledge is a necessary principle because apart from God's Word, society quickly spins into moral chaos without it. By educating ourselves about the types of cancer and the most common cancers, we can stay ahead of the game of health when it comes to prevention and detection.

One of the things you get from family, friends,

and colleagues when they know you have cancer, is how someone they know got rid of cancer and is living "cancer free." I have learned that even though we have the same cancer diagnosis, our treatments may be different because no two people experience cancer in the same way. But all treatments for cancer affect your daily life, at least for a time during and after treatments. A person can easily be overwhelmed by the decisions and choices that need to be made with healthcare providers, as well as communicating with family and friends about the services they want or can provide.

We have all been affected by Cancer. If you do not have cancer, you know someone, a friend or loved one who has cancer. Cancer dominates our society. It attacks our family, friends, and colleagues. A diagnosis of cancer is often a shock to the patient, family members, and friends. Some hear the diagnosis and manage to keep a positive attitude, find hope, and continue living their lives.

Others hear the diagnosis, and because there is no relationship with God, they have no hope and soon become depressed, and even suicidal. As a licensed professional counselor, I have helped clients deal with anxiety, denial, depression, hopelessness, and fear as a result of experiencing these trials in their life. Many of my clients are better able to cope once their treatment plan has been established and they can look forward to recovery.

The information in this book serves as the spiritual treatment plan toward recovery from the diagnosis of cancer. It was my experience as a counselor that helped me to avoid the denial and depression but, I could not help being "shocked" by the diagnosis: "You have Cancer." It was as if the doctor took out a gun and shot me in the head because your first thought is "I am dying." I realize this is a typical reaction to the diagnosis of cancer. It was my relationship with God that gave me hope and relieved my fear which allowed me to have a positive attitude about living with cancer realizing that God is a healer and He knows my future.

# CHAPTER 4:
# ROUTINE CHECKUP

*An annual checkup is a lifeline to early detection.*

I t all started with a routine checkup. I went to the doctor for my routine checkup in July 2011. There was no reason to suspect that my checkup would be anything other than "routine." I have always watched my nutrition and exercised at the YMCA two to three days per week. I do not have diabetes, high blood pressure, high cholesterol, or any other diseases that many people have.

I considered myself to be healthy and was shocked to receive a call from my Primary Care Physician. I received the bad news while attending my husband's family reunion in Huntsville, Alabama. My PCP told me that she had scheduled me to see an oncologist because of the findings from my blood sample. She said that the results from my blood work indicated mild anemia and an elevated protein level.

I kept my appointment with the oncologist, and he scheduled me for a bone marrow test in August which came back positive for cancer. My cancer diagnosis was Smoldering Multiple Myeloma. Myeloma is detected in the bone marrow.

Whether you have been diagnosed with cancer or are scheduling your doctor's appointment, I hope it gives you some relief to know that you are not alone. All cancers Matter to God. This is the time for you to seek Him for His healing power and put your trust in Him.

I will witness to His healing power as a result of my cancer journey while smoldering in the wilderness for almost five years. One night after discovering I could not raise myself out of bed, I was scheduled for an MRI. The MRI revealed that my cancer was not only active but had taken me to Mount Metastasis and attacked my cervix and spine. That was the beginning of my pain and anguish from the disease.

Radiation treatments were ordered in November to get me through the Thanksgiving holidays, and Chemotherapy began immediately after the holidays. I suffered from side effects of the chemo and was hospitalized in December. It was in the hospital that I witnessed a miraculous healing and realized that God keeps his promises.

The event which occurred during my hospital stay is one that has changed my life. When I look back and see where God has brought me from, I see that I have had things happen in my life that I never expected. God has blessed me beyond all measure. I will go further into detail when I share my ordeal in the Emergency Room which landed me a hospital stay.

# CHAPTER 5:
# THE DOCTOR'S
# APPOINTMENT

*Know the value of a companion when visiting the doctor.*

I never will forget the day I told my best girl-friend, Dr. Joyce Hardaway, that the doctor had diagnosed me with Cancer. She remarked about how athletic I was from regularly attending the YMCA and riding my bike. She observed how careful I was about my diet and sweets. She assumed it was breast cancer, but I told her it was Multiple Myeloma. She wanted to know just what the doctor said, so I explained to her that MM is a disease of the blood plasma. It was detected in my bone marrow, and there is no known cause and no known cure for it. He said it is a rare cancer and fewer than 200,000 people in the U.S. are diagnosed with it each year.

When I told Joyce, I had a follow-up appointment to see the doctor she asked if she could go with me as an extra set of ears. I know now the value of taking a companion with you for your follow-up appointments with the doctor, and I readily agreed. She did a little research on Myeloma and had formulated some questions to ask the doctor, to learn more about the disease. Her first question was "What is Multiple Myeloma?" The doctor explained that Multiple Myeloma is a type of cancer that affects plasma cells. Plasma cells are the white blood cells that make antibodies. Multiple Myeloma causes groups of abnormal plasma cells to accumulate in the bones. This can lead to the development of bone lesions. Abnormal plasma cells can also congregate in the bone marrow. Since bone marrow is the source of the body's blood cells, this interferes with the production of blood cells.

My friend made notes of the doctor's explanation. Before my annual checkup, I had not had any discomfort, pain or signs of any illness, so my next question was "what are the symptoms of MM?" The doctor went on to say that symptoms of myeloma vary from person to person. Initially, symptoms may not be noticeable. However, as the disease progresses, most patients will experience at least one of four major types of symptoms. These symptoms are generally referred to using the acronym CRAB. CRAB stands for Calcium, Renal, Anemia, and Bone damage. Other symptoms may include loss of appetite, bone pain, and fever.

I was told that I had Indolent Myeloma which had no current discernible symptoms. Indolent was the stage of my cancer. The stage of cancer is a summary of how far it has spread. It helps with predicting outcomes and in deciding what treatment is required. I asked about the treatment needed. The doctor said treatments include medications, chemotherapy, corticosteroids, radiation, or a stem-cell

> The words "YOU HAVE CANCER" were devastating and hard to acknowledge.

transplant. Joyce wrote all the information down, went home to google each treatment, and texted me a copy.

There are stages of the illness; my stage was "Smoldering." I asked the doctor if there was anything I could do, and he said nothing now, but come in for regular blood tests to follow the progression of the disease and be ready for treatment. When my girlfriend asked about treatment, the doctor suggested we just keep watch of the progression. When it was appropriate, we would discuss possible means of treating the disease.

I was glad my friend had gone with me to the doctor. We both talked positively about how we would just put our trust in God and pray for His healing power to cure me. God is still in the healing business, and He is looking for testimonies of those he saved in the flesh with the hopes of having them serve him. Those of us who have been saved must give light to the fact that he is Immanuel (God with Us). He still heals us just as He healed the woman with the issue of blood, the blind man, and the man with Leprosy. He even raised Lazarus from the dead. His healing powers still prevail for believers who trust and have Faith in Him.

The words "YOU HAVE CANCER" were devastating and hard to acknowledge. When the doctor made the announcement, I said, "Oh my God, what can I do?" It was if someone had taken a gun and shot me dead because to have cancer, which is incurable, ultimately means death. The doctor explained that there was nothing I could do other than get my blood checked every three months so that we can see the progression of cancer. Thoughts flooded my mind. I promised myself to pray, eat better, and exercise more, even though I already have a healthy lifestyle.

There is a benefit in taking a companion: your spouse, a relative or friend along with you to the doctor's office when going to get test results. When I cannot take a companion, I ask the doctor if I can tape the consultation. Dr. Jagasia is so competent with his practice as an oncologist and stem cell transplant specialist, he agrees. I tape our sessions so that I can listen to them later.

When I get home, my caregivers ask, "What did the doctor say?" I share the taped session with my immediate family which allows us all to be knowledgeable about my treatment. Thanks to Vanderbilt's online health connection at MyHealth @Vanderbilt.com, I can text any questions that arise and get a response. If it is not too urgent, I make a note of it on my cell phone under my "Ask the Doctor" notes for my next visit. My family feels more involved with my care because of these taped sessions.

# CHAPTER 6:
# LESSONS LEARNED IN
# THE VALLEY

*Trust in God with all your heart and lean not to thy own understanding.*

*(Proverbs 3:5)*

## 1. I Learned to Trust God

It was during my five years of smoldering that God molded me for the trials suffered in the Valley of the Shadow of Cancer. He sifted me, shaped me and taught me how to put my Trust in Him. God gave me a thirst to meditate on His Word. He connected me with the Holy Spirit, taught me the Impact of Prayer, and led me to His Healing Promises.

It is important to Listen, TRUST and Obey God. I cannot trust God if I am not in touch with Him. This is the scripture which gave me the idea that if I align with God, He will give me what I need and keep me on the right path to healing.

*Trust in the Lord and do good. Then you will live safely in the land and prosper. Take delight in the Lord, and he will give you your heart's desires. Commit everything you do to the LORD. Trust him, and he will help (heal) you. (Psalm 37:3-5)*

We align ourselves with our parents by obeying them. The same goes for alignment with God. We must obey his laws. When we are aligned with His will, our Father will give us our heart's desires—in His time. As we learn to enjoy Him for who He is, our (selfishness) self-focused wants are replaced by His perfect will and purpose for us.

When I commit my ways to God, I allow my thoughts, goals, and lifestyle to be shaped by His will and the things He loves. In other words, I acknowledge His right to determine whether my longing fits His plan. If I rest in the Lord and wait patiently for Him, then I will rely on Him to work out circumstances, even when the desire He has given me seems impossible. When

> **When circumstances are beyond my control, what I really believe will surface.**

He is my first love, my heart becomes focused on making His glory known in my life and trusting Him with my life in times of trials in the wilderness of brokenness and the Valley of the Shadow of Cancer.

When life gets hard, I used to get upset and wonder how long before the difficulty ends. I have learned that God wants me to focus on Him and not cancer. As I do this, I discover that He is doing essential spiritual work during my journey with cancer and other trials in my life.

I soon learned after studying God's word that what I needed to know about my life in Christ is spelled out in the BIBLE (Basic Instructions Before Leaving Earth). When circumstances are beyond my control, what I really believe will surface. The depth of my faith in God's character and promises becomes evident, as will any doubts or uncertainties I may have. For example, Joseph revealed strong belief and trust in God when he acknowledged that God intended his hardships for his good (Genesis 50:20 KJV)). You see, the enemy intended to harm me or break my spirit with cancer, but God intended it all for good. He brought me to this position so I can encourage and empower the lives of many people, including cancer victims. (Gen. 50:20 paraphrased)

If I do not trust God, I may find myself like Peter, denying him. There have been times when I did not succeed, the same as Peter, whose fear led him not to deny Christ, but to seek His presence. (John 18:25-27) Now I stop and think of trials as opportunities to grow, deepen my trust and faith in God. I had no fear of death or dying when I built a right relationship with God. I realized that death is eternal life with Him. I have no need to be fearful for I know Him and trust Him with my life.

Now because of the things I have learned from meditating on God's word, a cancer diagnosis would not be as devastating. I believe His promise of life eternal in the Kingdom. Readers who encounter trials may not be so devastated after reading this and gaining knowledge from my experience with cancer.

Do you want to know why I can trust God? I trust God because He loves me unconditionally. I will follow him anywhere knowing that he cares for me and loved me enough to give His life for my salvation. He died for me, and there is no greater love than His love for me.

Once I put my total trust in God, I found myself praying:

*Heavenly Father, you have brought me to the beginning of a new day. As the world is renewed fresh and clean, so I ask you to renew my heart with your strength and purpose. Forgive me the errors of yesterday and bless me to walk closer in your way today. This is the day I begin my life anew; shine through me so that every person I meet may feel your presence in my soul. Take my hand, precious Lord, for I cannot make it by myself. Through Christ, I pray and live. These things I ask in the mighty name of Jesus and by the authority of the Holy Spirit and the testimony of your Word to declare your works. Amen*

I used to think that life was hills and valleys when you go through a dark time, then I got to the mountaintop and had to travel down the valley of near death. I learned that it was my trust that gave me the faith in God to battle Cancer and led me out of the valley to Remission and into the Promised Land of Restoration.

## 2. I Learned to Meditate on God's Word

*He sent His Word, and healed them, and delivered them from their destructions. (Psalm 107:20)*

GOD'S WORD is my anchor and served a vital part of my life in the Valley of the Shadow of Cancer.

God's Word is not only the foundation for healing; it is the most powerful means to help me overcome discouragement. Whenever I started feeling down, I would reach for my Bible and turn to my favorite passage, Psalm 42:5. "Why are you in despair, O my soul?" As a counselor, I know that this question is the first step in overcoming discouragement. When we know why, we discover the cause and can plan to overcome. The Word has taught me that I am striving to be like Christ. He was an overcomer. He overcame the flesh, the World, and the devil. When I think of His life and how He took on humanity to model pain and suffering, I can overcome because I will never endure the pain or suffering that Christ had to endure and that comforts me.

Jesus is the Lord of my life. Sickness and disease have no power over me. I am forgiven and free from SIN AND GUILT. I am dead to sin and alive unto righteousness. (Colossians 1:21-22)

*Meditate on God's Word to Overcome Discouragement about Sickness:*

*Father, because of Your Word I am an over-comer of the devil, by the Blood of the Lamb and the word of my testimony.*

When you leave the doctor's office feeling discouraged behind that cancer diagnosis, look within. Before you can deal with your despair, you need to know what is causing it. Because you know the cause is cancer, you are ready to ask the Lord to help you on your journey and to heal you with His Word. I received the healing scriptures, and they were uplifting during my period of devastation. Cancer victims often are so devastated, they become depressed. I hope that my journey will empower you to have a positive attitude and know that God is a healer for those who obey him and put their trust in Him. We also must be patient and realize that God heals in His own time. I am still waiting and already claiming my healing because I learned that I must speak my healing as if it has already happened. This is what gives me hope and allows me to stay focused so that I can look up, look back and look to handle my discouragement that the diagnosis of cancer can bring.

**Look up** - I do this when I lift my eyes to the Lord and place my hope in Him. Remember, discouragement comes to everybody at one time or another, but it does not have to stay. In time, I shall again praise Him for the help of His presence. He was always there for he said, He would never leave me or forsake me. He was there in the Emergency Room and the Intensive Care Unit.

**Look back** - Despair has a way of erasing my memory of all the good the Lord has done for me over the years. Instead of wallowing in my present misery, I learned I must endeavor to remember His past care and provision. Then my faith will overpower cancer.

**Look Ahead** - Know that God's plan is to prosper me. "For I know the plans I have for you," (Jeremiah 29:11) So declares the Lord, as He plans to prosper me and not harm me, plans to give me hope and a future. I can look past cancer to what He is going to do in the future. He revealed that I will declare His works. His loving kindness will support me by day and bring comfort by night as I trust Him to work all things out for my good.

God's word is the foundation for healing. God has chosen me to live with a cancer diagnosis. I must give it my best. I will magnify and praise the

Lord, and He will use me to showcase His Love, grace, and mercy. I hope that this enlightenment will magnify the LORD and reach out to all those who are trying to find answers dealing with trials including cancer.

I learned that it was God's Word that would allow me to develop my relationship with Him, so I learned to meditate on the scriptures (His Word) and Walk with Him daily. Even when I feel lonely, I am never alone.

When my focus is right, I can respond correctly in spite of my trial with cancer. I can declare the Works of the LORD when I fix my eyes on the Lord. Circumstances and the devil may cause me to think He's forgotten about me, but His Word promises that He's there and will bring me through this journey with cancer. Dr. Charles Stanley's "Life Principles" reminds me to Obey God and leave all the consequences to Him.

## 3. I Learned the Holy Spirit Intercedes for Me in Times of Trouble

God speaks by the Holy Spirit through the Bible meditation, prayer, circumstances, and the church to reveal Himself, His purposes and His Ways to bring us comfort in times of sickness and trials in life.

Holy Spirit is the third person of the Trinity.

He awaits us to ask for help in times of trials. The Spirit of the Lord is upon me because he anointed me to declare His Works. "He has commissioned me to proclaim release to the captives of Cancer and recovery of sickness and disease, to set free those who are oppressed, to proclaim the favorable works of the Lord." The Holy Spirit revealed, *"You will not die but live to declare the Works of God." (Psalm 118:17)*

I work hard to stay plugged into God so that the Holy Spirit can intercede for me. It is important if I am going to communicate my needs and desires through prayer. Think of this scenario: God talks to us through the Holy Spirit so that we can let our light shine for Him. When we fail to focus on Him each day, we become unplugged, and our lights are like those hidden under a bush. When we are unplugged, He cannot communicate with us. I am thankful that He is sovereign and knows all about my needs and desires.

I stay plugged in so that I can ASK: says, "Ask whatever you need, seek and you shall find, knock and the door will be open to you." (Matthew 7:7)

*A- ASK Him for my healing and any other thing I need or want,*

*S- SEEK Him so that I can find answers about cancer and His Promises*

*K- KNOCK so that He can open the door of my heart to come in, comfort me and keep me from being lonely or feeling all alone.*

We are filled with the Spirit! The Holy Spirit came into my heart when I decided to give my life to Christ, to become a Christian at age six. I continually ASK the Holy Spirit to lead me, to guide me, to help me do the things God wants me to do. I learned in the hospital that my growth allowed me to let the Holy Spirit take control. According to John 14, it was the Holy Spirit which allowed me to be

> **I used to find myself too busy to entertain the Holy Spirit.**

comforted by the 23rd Psalm. He became my "Counselor" to guide me in my everyday life. The Spirit works through my conscience to make me aware of sin in my life. It convicts me of my sins. It knows what and how to pray when I have no clue.

The Holy Spirit taught me the importance of Hope and believing God for His promises. Abraham was a man of faith, and he went up the mountain with Isaac, his son, willing to sacrifice him. All the while, he was hoping for an intervention from God. Abraham's story empowered me to believe that God will bring me a miraculous healing if I exemplify the faith of Abraham. I hope that God has full control and that I can accept His will. I desire to live longer in the flesh here on earth to declare His works before accepting death as eternal life if it is His Will.

I used to find myself too busy to entertain the Holy Spirit. I think of my connection with the Holy Spirit as Christ's light that shines in me. Just as light will not shine in a lamp that is not plugged in or filled with oil, I must pray and meditate daily to make sure I am plugged into God. He communicates to me through the Holy Spirit, and I communicate with Him through prayer and meditation. John teaches us that Christ on the day of Pentecost left the Holy Spirit as our comforter and the 23rd Psalm comforts us in times of trouble and trials.

Yea, though I walk through the Valley of the Shadow of Death, I was fearful in the ER (emergency room). Once I felt the presence of the Holy Spirit, I overcame the mixture of my emotions of fear and anger at God for encouraging me to take that Chemo.

Daily I rejoice and praise God for protection and salvation from devastating side effects. I share my voice of thanksgiving for God's miraculous provision, for His prevailing grace in the early discovery of my metastasis, for His incredible power in the hospital when my vitals failed and became unstable. Over and over, I have been favored by the miraculous acts of His kindness. I know what it is like to feel the comfort of God because of the Holy Spirit.

King David knew what it was like to experience God's comfort and protection. He knew what it meant to walk through the valley of the shadow of death. He knew where to turn in times of sorrow and grief. In one of the most memorized passages of scripture in the Bible, David wrote his very personal Psalm of comfort, hope, and promise.

> *"The Lord is my shepherd; I shall not want. He maketh me to lie down in green pastures: he leadeth me beside the still waters. He restoreth my soul: he leadeth me in the paths of righteousness for his name's sake. Yea, though I walk through the valley of the shadow of death, I will fear no evil: for thou art with me; thy rod and thy staff they comfort me. Thou preparest a table before me in the presence of mine enemies: thou anoints my head with oil; my cup runs over. Surely goodness and mercy shall follow me all the days of my life: and I will dwell in the house of the Lord forever."*
> *(Psalm 23)*

## 4. I Learned These Healing Scriptures During My Walk with God

### *Exodus 15:26*

*He said, "If you listen carefully to the Lord your God and do what is right in his eyes, if you pay attention to his commands and keep all his decrees, I will not bring on you any of the diseases I brought on the Egyptians, for I am the LORD, who heals you."*

### *1 Peter 2:24*

*He himself bore our sins" in his body on the cross, so that we might die to sins and live for righteousness; "by his wounds you have been healed.*

### *James 5:14*

*Is anyone among you sick? Let them call the elders of the church to pray over them and anoint them with oil in the name of the LORD?*

### *Proverbs 4:20-22*

*My son, pay attention to what I say; turn your ear to my words. Do not let them out of your sight; keep them within your heart; for they are life to those who find them and health to one's whole body.*

### Psalm 107:19-21

*Then they cried to the LORD in their trouble, and he saved them from their distress. He sent His word and healed them; he rescued them from the grave. Let them give thanks to the LORD for his unfailing love and his wonderful deeds for mankind.*

### Exodus 23:25

*Worship the LORD your God and his blessing will be on your food and water. I will take away sickness from among you.*

### Psalm 30:2

*Lord my God, I called to you for help, and you healed me.*

### Isaiah 53:4-5

*Surely, he took up our pain and bore our suffering, yet we considered him punished by God, stricken by him, and afflicted. But he was pierced for our transgressions, he was crushed for our iniquities; the punishment that brought us peace was on him, and by his wounds we are healed.*

### Psalm 103:2-3

*Praise the LORD, my soul, and forget not all his benefits. God forgives all our sins, heals all our diseases, and who redeems our life from the pit and crowns us with love and compassion.*

### Psalm 41:3

*The LORD sustains them on their sickbed and restores them from their bed of illness.*

### Psalm 147:3

*He heals the brokenhearted and binds up their wounds.*

### Jeremiah 17:14

*Heal me, LORD, and I will be healed; save me and I will be saved, for you are the one I praise.*

### Psalm 103:2-5

*Let all that I am praise the LORD, may I never forget the good things he does for me. He forgives all sins and heals all my diseases. He redeems me from death and crowns me with love and tender mercies. He fills my life with good things. My mouth is renewed like the eagles!*

### Psalm 91:10-11

*If you say, "The Lord is my refuge, and you make the Most High your dwelling, no harm will overtake you, no disaster (or cancer) will come near your tent.*

### Proverbs 12:28

*In the way of righteousness there is life; along*

*that path is immortality. (The way of the godly leads to life not death.)*

### Matthew 8:17

*This was to fulfill what was spoken through the prophet Isaiah: "He took up our infirmities and bore our diseases." (He took our sickness and removed our disease according to Isaiah 53:5)*

### John 6:63

*The Spirit gives eternal life and Human effort accomplishes nothing. The very words I have spoken to you are Spirit and life.*

### Galatians 3:13

*Christ redeemed us from the curse of the law... (Christ has rescued me from the curse pronounced by law. When He was hung on the cross, He took the curse for our wrongdoing upon himself.)*

### Mark 11:23

*Truly I tell you, if anyone says to this mountain, 'Go, throw yourself into the sea,' and does not doubt in their heart but believes that what they say will happen, it will be done for them. (You can say to this mountain be lifted up and thrown into the sea, but nothing will happen unless you truly believe.)*

## Luke 17:6

*If I have faith as small as a mustard seed, I can demand or command my health, and it would obey me.*

## Romans 12:1-2

*And so, dear brothers and sisters, I plead with you to give your bodies to God because of all he has done for you. Let them be a living and holy sacrifice the kind he will find acceptable. This is truly the way to worship him. Do not copy the behavior and customs of this world, but let God transform you into a new person by changing the way you think. Then you will learn to know God's will for you, that is good and pleasing and perfect.*

## John 14:20

*On that day (When I am resurrected), you will know that I am in my Father and you are in me, and I am in you.*

How can you tell if you are being led by the Spirit? You can tell by the "fruit" of your life—your attitudes and actions. "The fruit of the Spirit is love, joy, peace, patience, kindness, goodness, faithfulness, gentleness, and self-control." (Galatians 5:22-23) These are the Christ-like characteristics that keep me in step with the Spirit.

Jesus says, He no longer calls me his servant but calls me His friend. As said in John 15:15, talking with God develops a deeper relationship with Him.

## 5. I Learned Prayer Is Spending Time Talking with God.

Prayer can be a form of religious practice, either individual or communal and can take place in public or in private. It may involve the use of words, song, or complete silence. When we speak a prayer, it may be in the form of a hymn, a formal creed statement, or a spontaneous utterance or in tongues from the person praying. There are different kinds of prayer. There is the petitioner's prayer, a petition that requests and commonly addressed to a government official or public entity. We have the prayer of supplication, thanksgiving, and praise.

Take the opportunity to spend time with God in prayer and remember all you need to do is ASK the LORD for help and pray. Be guided in your prayer with the ACTS. My prayers are usually tailored by this acronym ACTS:

**A - Adoration,**
**C - Confession**
**T - Thanksgiving**
**S - Supplication**

It is my (A C T S) that seeks to activate a rapport with God to reverence Him through deliberate communication. Prayer is an action word.

*I adore you, LORD, because you are worthy to be praised. Please forgive me as I confess my Sins whether they were sins of omission or commission. Father, I come with thanksgiving in my heart. Thanking you for the many trials you have brought me through safely and once more Father, I bow in supplication and ask that you hear my prayer.*

*(ACTS of prayer)*

This acronym guides me to make sure I am giving Him the highest Adoration or praise, being repentant of and confessing my sins, for we all sin and come short of the glory of God. I always give him Thanks for the many blessings He bestows upon me and then I can pray in Supplication, pleading humbly to communicate the needs or desires of my heart. When I put this into action, my prayer would emerge.

---

**Prayer is the act to reconnect with Jesus Christ.**

---

Cancer changed everything including my workday schedule as a Licensed Professional Counselor. The one thing that did not change was my early morning devotional time. It is still at 5:00 a.m. because my earliest chemotherapy treatments are not scheduled before 7:30 a.m. and my labs may start as early as 7:00 a.m. This is the time of morning when the cell phone is silent, the house is quiet, the birds are not singing, and there is little traffic noise. This is an excellent time for uninterrupted Prayer and devotion.

I was amazed at how God knew how to refer my clients to meet my treatment schedule. I usually get random referrals. I soon realized that these referrals are truly the people God sent to counseling for me to care for through leadership of the Holy Spirit. Christian counseling forms a triangle of support which consists of the client, the counselor, and the Holy Spirit.

Whenever we experience sickness, our first step is to pray and ask the Lord how He wants us to respond. He may tell us to trust Him for healing, or He may want us to seek counseling and medical help. I thought of Paul who did both. It was the scriptures about Paul that started me believing that God might choose to heal me through a physician. Remember, Paul sought healing from the Lord, trusted God's choice for his life, and relied on Luke's help in times of suffering. My goal was to be God-conscious, realizing that the One who saved Paul is walking with me through this valley of smoldering and brokenness. God will direct my steps when I keep my mind on Him. Prayer is an action word. Continuous Prayer is the simplest way to stay focused on God.

Prayer is the act to reconnect with Jesus Christ. Our relationship with God was broken, apart from Jesus Christ. When Adam and Eve rebelled, their nature became corrupt and alienated them from God. That "flesh" nature was then passed down to all subsequent generations, separating us from the Father. When Adam sinned, sin entered the world. Adam's sin brought death, so death spread to everyone for, everyone has sinned as written in (Romans 5:12). On my own, I can neither make amends for my sin nor change my nature. I can align myself with His commands and character.

I must pray and meditate daily to make sure I am aligned with God. I realize that I am going to have hard times in life and my life will be met with trials and tribulations of the fallen world and that is why I must go to the Lord in prayer.

God allows me to be His greatest passion because I am a believer struggling to live my life aligned with His. I say struggling because the flesh is weak and the enemy preys on our weakness. Because I love the Lord, I rely on His strength for my connection with Him. He has priority over my possessions, vocation, and even other relationships. When I find myself not focusing on God and becoming anxious or fixed on an outcome, I begin to pray for realignment.

It is in the prayer of alignment that helped me realize that I am to delight in the LORD which means to take pleasure in discovering more about Him and following His will. I received my diagnosis, decided to seek God's protection, and was reminded to put on the whole armor of God.

Prayer changed me, and prayer changes things. My Aunt, Elizabeth Finley, survived many physical calamities including a gunshot wound. She gave me a prayer for health and healing when I told her I had been diagnosed with cancer. I wish I knew where this prayer came from so I could give it reference. My Aunt got it from her mother, Daisy Finley. She is deceased. This prayer reads as follows:

> "Father, in the name of Jesus, I confess
> Your Word concerning healing. As I do
> this, I believe and say that Your Word will
> not return to you void, but will accomplish
> what it says it will. Therefore, I believe in

the name of Jesus that I am healed according to the scripture 1 Peter 2.24. It is written in Your Word that Jesus Himself took my infirmities and bore my sicknesses according to the scripture Matthew 8:17. Therefore, with great boldness and confidence, I say on the authority of the written Word that I am redeemed from the curse of sickness, and I refuse to tolerate its symptoms.

Satan, I speak to you in the name of Jesus and say that your principalities, powers, your master spirits who rule the present darkness and your spiritual wickedness in heavenly places are bound from operating against me in any way. I am loosed from your assignment. I am the property of Almighty God, and I give you no place in me. I dwell in the secret place of the Most High God, I abide, remain stable and fixed under the shadow of the Almighty, whose power no foe can withstand.

Now, Father, because I reverence and worship you, I have the assurance of Your Word that the angel of the Lord encamps around about me and delivers me from every evil work. No evil shall befall me, no plague or calamity shall come near my dwelling. I confess the word of God abides in me and delivers to me perfect soundness of mind and wholeness in body and spirit from the deepest parts of my nature in my immortal spirit even to the joints and marrow of my bones. That Word is medication and life to my flesh."

In emergencies, prayer gives me clear guidance and eliminates confusion. When I read and heard about the side effects of Chemo, I immediately sought the Lord through fasting and prayer. I began to think He may want me to seek medical help. Despite His power, Jesus did not heal every sick person in Israel. When He visited His hometown, He could not perform many miracles because of the people's unbelief. We also live in a society that doubts Jesus' ability to heal. God is my healer, and I encourage you to believe the same.

Now, I have on the whole armor of God, and the shield of faith protects me from all the fiery darts of Satan. Cancer taught me that Jesus is the High Priest of my confessions, and I hold fast to my confession of faith in His Word. I stand immovable and fixed in full assurance that I have health and healing NOW in the name of Jesus.

I prayed and prayed and waited on the LORD for a miraculous healing. I waited five years for that miraculous healing before God miraculously raised me up from a deadly viral infection during my struggle with side effects of radiation and chemotherapy. I am a firm believer and witness that prayer works. Prayer leads us to our desire and calls for devotion to God.

Prayer is what brought me peace and allowed me to refocus on Him when I felt all alone in the Emergency Room. God's Word says: Prayer will produce peacefulness when we begin each day with God, He will help us remain calm and feel tranquil.

*Peace I leave with you; my peace I give to you. Not as the world gives do I give to you. Let not your hearts be troubled, neither let them be afraid. (John 14:27)*

## 6. I Learned to Stand on God's Promises

Once I learned to trust God, I began dwelling on the promises of His word. When you continually dwell on thoughts of His victory, favor, faith, power, and strength, nothing can hold you back (Deuteronomy 31:1). The promises God communicated to me were:

1. *Trust in the Lord with all your heart, and lean not on your own understanding; in all your ways acknowledge Him, and He shall direct your paths.* (Proverbs 3:5-6)

*2. Jesus answered them. "Destroy this temple, and I will raise it again in three days." (John 2:19)*

*3. You will not die but live to declare the Works of the LORD. (Psalm 118:17)*

I adopted these promises after receiving my diagnosis and decided to live my life to the fullest. To the fullest meant not canceling any of the activities I already had planned.

There were three pressing activities on my calendar while I was yet smoldering with cancer. When I received my diagnosis in July 2011, I already had plans to go to Jerusalem in November of that same year. God really does know my future because the trip to the Holy Land was just the thing I needed to give me a better Hope. While in Jerusalem, I went to the Western Wall, also called the Wailing Wall, and there I wrote my prayer request that God would take on my battle with cancer and give me peace and victory over death.

Another activity was an arrangement to attend a Health Camp to learn all about healthy nutrition. While attending the health camp, God revealed the Scripture informing me that, "I shall not die, but live, and declare the works of the Lord." (Psalm 118:17) The third activity was a trip to Jamaica. My husband John and I had plans to spend our forty-sixth anniversary in Jamaica. I felt God leading me to seek a healthier lifestyle after He led me to the Seventh Day Adventist environment. It was in that environment that I learned about the health camp and vegan diet.

I wanted to go to Jamaica before attending the health camp so I could enjoy the Jamaican cuisine without feeling guilty about my choice of food. I rescheduled the health camp activity to follow our anniversary. So that meant postponing the health camp and enrolling in the next program which did not start until September. At this point, I was still controlling things; meaning, I was not operating from my trust in God. I was my controlling self. I called and changed the date to allow my trip to Jamaica first.

When I first started this journey, God had me examine myself. He revealed that I was self-centered and not God-centered. The rubric against which I was evaluated was the "Christ-like Characteristics" found in Galatians 20. Even though I could claim all of them in some respect, God had me realize that I did things on my own and did them my way. He called that control or "controlling matters." He pointed out the confidence I had in thinking I was following His lead was pride simply because I could not be in control and follow at the same time. Once God finished with my "examination of self" I began to change my actions and behavior to keep from conflicting with God's plans for me. I wanted to respect His will for my life.

I felt God had taken me to the Promised Land. The trip to Jamaica was like Heaven on Earth. It was truly my walk with God during that time that caused me to wait for His healing. I was looking for a miraculous cure after smoldering for five years. I waited and waited for God's healing and assumed it would miraculously come over time and all the while I know that I was presumptuous in what I expected from the Lord. For example, the doctor wanted to start treatment in October 2015, and because I was still waiting on my miraculous cure, I tried to hold off longer. I was so presumptuous I could not follow His lead until I adopted "Trust in the Lord." (Proverbs 3:5)

I adopted this as my daily scripture. It was my family; a devoted husband, daughter, son, and nephew who assured me that God allows medical physicians to perform His miracles too. Someone said the doctor's hands are His hands of healing here on earth. I was praying and fasting, fasting and praying when the Holy Spirit revealed that the physician had already been chosen and named by a former student of mine, Dr. Sunil S. Geevarghese. I remembered calling Sunil to ask him to recommend a good oncologist at Vanderbilt where he works. God blessed me with a network of former students in all walks of life. Dr. Geevarghese is a transplant surgeon. He referred me to Dr. Madan Jagasia in 2011 who has monitored my smoldering for five years.

My October 2015 visit should have been the appointment to start my treatment. The doctor, aware of my hope in Jesus, said that my numbers were compliant with the new guidelines for treatment, but since I wasn't a new patient and knowing my history, he would wait for the flu-like symptoms. I was operating on the fact that God had broken me, taught me many things about healing, and left me smoldering so that He could cure me any day now. I accepted the delay of treatment. I was leaning towards my own understanding. I don't do that now for I adopted this scripture to guard against doing things my way.

## My favorite scripture:

*Trust in the Lord with all your heart and lean not to thy own understanding but, acknowledge Him and He will direct your path. (Proverbs 3:5-6)*

This scripture is necessary for me because I was raised by my mother and grandmother, two strong-willed women who modeled control and decision-making plans. I had to learn that God was in control, not me. I had to be careful not to control things after giving them to God. I would pray and ask for God's direction but, when the enemy (Satan) would cause doubt in my mind by saying, "God gave you five senses, so do you think He wants you to just sit here and wait, or have you help yourself? Why don't you pick up that phone and call..." Satan would have me thinking, "Who do they think they are?"

When he prompted me in this way normally, I would respond by modeling the control I had seen modeled growing up. It was during my devotions, my close walk and talk with God that He reminded me of His sovereignty over Satan and that when I surrender things to Him and have faith that He will take care of me and provide for me. I have read in His word that His word does not come back void. Proverbs 4:22 tells us that God's words are life to us and medicine to all our flesh. Today, I feel like an overcomer. I have overcome the world, the flesh, and Satan. I have learned to put all my trust in God Almighty.

God's second promise was about the Chemo that was delivered to my house, before my treatment. I had bad vibes, call it intuition or whatever.

I call it discernment of the Holy Spirit. I felt convicted that the chemo was not going to be good for me. I laid the package of chemo on the altar, and I began to pray seeking God's will for me and the chemotherapy. Each day I looked at the package on the altar, and I would pray. One Sabbath morning the Holy Spirit spoke with this scripture:

*Jesus answered them. "Destroy this temple, and I will raise it again in three days." (John 2:19)*

I did not grasp a meaning for this scripture at first. God needed to get my attention, and so He did. He broke me! I was lost in the valley of brokenness and wondering "why me Lord?" It was in the valley that God educated me about His word, the Holy Spirit, His healing Scriptures, the impact of prayer and the importance of trust and faith in Him. It was a quiet Sabbath morning that this scripture revealed itself to me. If the chemo destroys me, God will raise me up in three days. I was confused thinking I had to die to be raised in three days. I was really confused because He gave me the following scripture:

*You will not die but live to declare the work of the LORD. (Psalm 118:17)*

This scripture was an eye-opener. The Holy Spirit revealed it to me during my stay at the health camp, MEET Ministries (Missionary Education & Evangelistic Training) located in Huntington, Tennessee. This is where the Holy Spirit revealed the scripture. I liked what it said for it uplifted my spirit and I shared it with the others attending the Bible study that afternoon. We all took turns giving meaning to it. This scripture needed no explanation. It was as plain as the noses on my face. It meant God truly had something for me to do and that I was going to be spared to fulfill His purpose. It also gave clarity to John 2:19. If my temple is destroyed, I will not die. I became content with this promise. I do not want to die even though I know I will have eternal life in His Kingdom. I have always enjoyed serving God and pursuing His purpose for my life.

My co-author, MM Cancer, will share my smoldering days with you. I am grateful to MM for not attacking my organs for five years. His tour will take us smoldering through the valley of Brokenness, up the Mountain Top of Metastasis and down the Valley of Side Effects of the Shadow of Cancer. When he becomes too weak from the radiation and chemotherapy to continue, he relinquishes his fight. I, author Charlaine, will continue the tour, encountering the setbacks from the side effects ahead of the remission required

before going over into the Promised Land of Restoration.

# CHAPTER 7:
# THE CANCER SPEAKS

*The Smoldering Tour to
Mount Metastasis and Side Effects Valley.*

Welcome aboard folks! It's about time I was recognized. After all, there, would be no book if it were not for me. I would be the star character but, Cancer is no match for God.

## Smoldering Journey through the Valley from Cancer's Point of View

Wow, it is about time I had a say in this matter. My name is MM which stands for Multiple Myeloma, and I will be your tour guide during the smoldering stage. We will start in the Valley of Brokenness before climbing up Mt. Metastasis. Then, I will lead you through the Valley of Side Effects. Once we finish the side effects, my tour will end because the next stop is in the hospital and Charlaine will take over the Hospital Stay journey. She wants to make sure you see how fear takes over at the ER.

> I could tell early on that she planned on being an overcomer of cancer

Check me out! I'm a smoldering cancer named Multiple Myeloma. Some of the doctors and patients call me MM for short. Now that I have introduced the path, come on follow me.

I started out smoldering and smoldered in the wilderness for almost five years. I call this my "valley journey" because, after my attack on Charlaine's bone marrow in June 2015, I hung out in the blood while Charlaine learned lessons from God. He taught her many things. I never will forget how God sifted, shaped and molded her for His purpose. I remember her asking, "Why me LORD?" and God revealed to her that He wanted to use her talents. He wanted to draw her closer to Him. He wanted her to declare His healing message to others who are struggling with trials of life.

I could tell early on that she planned on being an overcomer of cancer. The days in the valley were long and tiring for me because I rested while Charlaine did all the work. She would wake me up some nights crying and questioning God. I wondered what the fuss was all about, after all, I am a nice guy. I know cancers that are so invasive they require immediate radiation or chemotherapy. I could have been more invasive, but I chose to smolder and give her time to seek God for the "miraculous cure" she was so sure she would get.

Each month she would drag me to Nashville for tests. The doctors would tell her that I was still there hanging out in the blood just smoldering. I call it "hanging out." I would sit around each day watching her pray, meditate, and study the scriptures. I got so tired of her bragging to her friends how much she was learning on her journey with cancer. She did not seem to mind how hard it was in the valley keeping up with her regular routine schedule and obeying God at the same time. God told her that she would wander around in the valley until she learned what He intended for her to know to overcome her cancer trial. Then she'd be ready to declare His Works in the Promise Land of Restoration.

The lessons stretched out over four-plus years. Well, at least she did not wander in the valley for as long as those Israelites wandered in the wilderness. They tell me they wandered in the wilderness for forty years. They could have reached the Promised Land in seven years, but I heard they did not obey God. Whew, forty years! I doubt I could hang out that long, but I would have, knowing that once I metastasized, they would try to kill me.

I had the doctor and Charlaine waiting on me almost five years before I got tired of the inactivity. That's when I decided to act out, so I didn't lose my freaking mind. I had her wondering if she truly had cancer. She couldn't feel me because I'd been kind enough to just smolder, and not use aches or pain.

Acting out meant metastasizing to an organ, and I guess the back was as good a place as any. At first, I did not know exactly where I wanted to start. The doctor had given her a hint that I would probably attack her somewhere in her back so I decided not to disappoint her. I gave her fair warning, but she tried to ignore me. One morning after she finished her meditation and began to stretch out on the floor, I poked her in her lower abdomen. Since the doctor had mentioned my attack zone would be in her back, she paid me no attention at all. I will not be ignored and thought, "Who does she think I am?"

The next day after her two-mile brisk walk, I jabbed her in a muscle in her back, and that got her attention. I jabbed her and immediately felt some restraint. It was the all-powerful God holding me back. I decided not to get into it with Him because He always wins. She told her son about the pain, and he thought she may be dealing with a pinched nerve instead of me, cancer MM.

The next week, I heard her and her husband discussing that trip to Jamaica again. They were all geared up to celebrate their forty-fifth anniversary. I thought, oh what the hell, I need a vacation myself. Lying around on the beach should be fun. No more attacks for now.

She told her daughter about plans to attend a missionary camp for a cleansing and lessons on God's Plan for Nutrition, Health, and Wellness. She told her daughter that she was delaying her cleanse until after her Jamaica trip so she would not feel guilty about eating. She said, "I want to be able to enjoy all the different cuisines including the jerk chicken, rum cake, and other favorite island recipes on my Jamaica Paradise trip." I watched her. She was all excited about going to Jamaica. She told her friends she had wanted to go to Jamaica ever since reading the book and watching the movie, "How Stella Got Her Groove Back."

After another two weeks of the regular routine, we arrived in Montego Bay, Jamaica. I thought to myself, they put a lot into this trip so I might as well behave and just enjoy myself. I am sure those Jamaican cuisines will be tasty. They will probably be full of fructose sugar, and the meats will have lots of fat. I love sweets. They help me thrive in the bloodstream.

I was hidden away smoldering while they enjoyed an all-inclusive stay at the Coyaba Bay Beach Resort. She would get up every morning and drag me out to the oceanfront and spend the entire day there relaxing in the lounge chaise while reading her Bible. She loved walking the beachside, water exercising and, of course, we all enjoyed eating at the different venues. I was glad she put off going to the nutrition camp because I heard you're only allowed to eat vegetables and maybe a little fruit. Hey, while in Jamaica, we ate hamburgers, hotdogs, French fries, fish, and jerk chicken. Her husband likes pork, and he enjoyed Bar-B-Que ribs.

The all-inclusive allowed them to eat as much as they wanted to eat, whenever they wanted to eat. I loved the sweet treats because cancer loves sweets and, of course, she does not know that yet, haha! I gave her a sweet craving that was out of this world. It made the whole trip worth my while.

Hey, I thought she came over here to Jamaica to get her groove back! I have watched her spend five amazing days here. She has been spending time studying and meditating on the Word at the ocean side while her husband snoozed to the sound of the waves. Unlike Stella, she has a husband. He is her groove.

Five days of enjoyment and now, Charlaine remembered her fifty percent off coupon for a Jamaican Massage. She began to think more and more about her Jamaican massage. You see, she was awarded a half off coupon for selecting the Honeymoon Suite. It was part of her Marriage celebration at their "all-inclusive stay" at Coyaba Beach in Montego Bay. Satan had her right where he wants her:

She was deceived by a false sense of reward. Three enemies are constantly at work trying to bring her down—namely the devil, his world system, and our own treacherous weak flesh, and oh yes, and MM Cancer. I cannot leave me out. Her celebration was ending, and she just couldn't leave the island without her "Jamaican Massage." She woke up on the sixth day with the massage on her mind when her mind should have been" stayed on Jesus." One thing I noticed on the valley journey is that whenever Charlaine woke up and got into her devotion, the enemy was no match for her because she was Christ-focused. But this day, Satan and the worldly focus had taken over. She was tempted and focused on that massage.

Satan knew that even though she'd have a righteous standing before God, she must, like Paul, acknowledge an internal problem: "sin which dwells in her" (Rom. 7:20). Satan took full advantage of this weakness, luring her with fleshly and worldly temptations. Her enemy, Satan stoked her pride, and she became unaware of her own vulnerability.

That day, she got up early looking for her coupon to get the massage and could not find it anywhere. She was getting frantic. She asked her husband to help her locate the coupon, and they both looked for it with no results. I was perfectly fine because I did not feel like being disturbed with all that pressing, pulling and rubbing. I was glad she could not find it. Well, she would not be outdone. She called down to the main desk to see if she could get the massage without the coupon.

She verified to the desk clerk her vacation package which included the honeymoon suite, oceanside balcony, champagne, flowers, chocolates, and a fifty percent off coupon for a Jamaican massage.

Thinking only of herself, Charlaine took full control, and the enemy was waiting because he knew instead of waking this morning with her focus on God, she was focused on that massage. I applauded God for purposely keeping her from finding the coupon because I did not want one but, she was so insistent and took the control from God with the enemy's help. She won the battle and got her massage without the coupon. I would have rather stayed on the oceanfront relaxing, but there I was being massaged.

The massage was vigorous, and there was a pop when the therapist stretched and extended her left arm forward. He said, "Oooh My, your joints are tight." She tipped the therapist and thought he had done a great job on tight muscles. Tight muscle or not it made just the right starting place for my metastasis to begin. I knew she would soon be in trouble. It was the massage that ushered the metastasis to her spine. A little late, but now she realizes that because Myeloma is a bone cancer, she should have been cautious of her weakening joints and bones. Her massage therapist at home in Chattanooga gave her gentle massages.

Their vacation ended on September 2nd. As they were boarding the plane to return to the States, I heard her tell her husband that she realizes now that God had her misplace the coupon to discourage her from getting the massage. You know, it is like the situation when you cannot find your car keys. You are sure it is God delaying you for your own good. Once she realized what happened, she started making sure that she woke each morning with her focus on Christ Jesus so that He could direct her day's activities. Now I know why, every morning, she religiously says, *"Trust in the Lord with all my heart and lean not to my own understanding; in all my ways submit to Him, and He will make my paths straight."* *(Proverbs 3:5-6)* It keeps her from being in control. Now, she is careful to follow God's lead.

Well, we will have a little break here before climbing up to Mt. Metastasis. I need to rest up for the attack. Attacking organs is tiring work because the Chemo tries to protect them from me.

## Mount Metastasis

### Myeloma attacks organs

The following week after returning from Jamaica, she went to the MEET (Missionary, Education & Evangelistic Training) Ministry mission home in Huntington, Tennessee. It's a multifaceted program providing a Home Natural Lifestyle Retreat. MEET's aim is to help revive True Medical Missionary Work, by educating and training consecrated Gospel-Medical Missionaries for the mission fields, and to establish missionary centers throughout the world.

Little did she know that I was active and about to make an attack on her organs. She was absorbed by the lessons about me (cancer) and how to cure herself with diet and natural herbs. I decided to wait around a little longer before attacking her spine, the area jeopardized during the massage. We spent two weeks there learning about cancer, nutrition, health, and wellness. They even had a large garden, a couple of green-houses, and taught her how to grow her own vegetables. She had to drink those nasty green juices four times a day. Boy, I hate that kale, parsley, carrots, and beet juice. There is not a bit of sweet flavor to them, and I do love sugary drinks. I would settle for an apple or some berries in that juice.

By the end of the two weeks, I was really craving something sweet, but, Charlaine had been cleansed of all the toxins and had no desire for sweets or meats. She had lost eleven pounds and had become accustomed to the diet they had prescribed for her. She had become a Vegetarian. She noticed a slight ache in her lower right side while exercising each morning. I wondered how long she would ignore me and keep quiet. She finally told her therapist at the camp about the ache. They used a charcoal poultice, wrapping her side so it could penetrate her liver and hip to alleviate the pain and clean the liver organ.

It was late October, and Charlaine was still following the vegetarian diet. She was still losing weight, so much weight that her family became concerned. I heard her son say, "Mom, now you need to eat something other than just those salads every day." I had made my attack and was not getting any sweets or meats.

She contacted her doctor via "Myhealthat-Vanderbilt.com" who wanted to wait and address it at her upcoming appointment. I asked myself, "Why won't she go now to the ER for tests?" I remembered she was still praying for God to heal her miraculously and believed that she would be healed. Charlaine learned that to hope is simply to dream. Hope constitutes dreams, prayers, and expectations and trying to give it all to God and let Him be in control. She waited and prayed, prayed and waited until the pain became unbearable.

My attack became more evident in early November when she tried to get out of bed one night and could not lift her body up to a sitting position. I said, "I guess you'll listen to MM now!" But, instead of going to the emergency room, she kept her appointment with her oncologist doctor at Vanderbilt that next day. I heard her doctor tell her that the cancer, that is me, was active and that she needed to start treatment now.

When we arrived back to Chattanooga, her first stop was at the ER because she felt her throat getting sore. Wow, when I got active and metastasized outside of the bone marrow, I could not stop just at the spine. Since the Jamaican massage damaged the thoracic T9 spine, I attacked it first, but then I attacked her vertebra, the C4. The enemy enticed me to attack the spine.

The devil had me to attack Charlaine's voice box, too. He, the enemy, remembered the Holy Spirit giving her that Psalm 118:17 at the missionary camp requesting that she Declare His Works. He wanted to destroy her voice so she would not be able to declare those Works of the LORD. Satan told me that he also did not want to hear any testimonies later about what God had done for her on her journey with cancer. He was using me to help block God's plan.

Well, here we are at the ER, heading up to the Mountaintop of Metastasis after smoldering all the way through the Jamaican trip. All I can say is that normally when I attack the spine, the person is not able to stand or stay upright without being in unbearable pain. Charlaine must have a guardian angel or someone taking care of her, because I kept hearing the X-ray technician say how remarkable, writing it up in his report. I believe that "remarkable" meant that the damage should have been a lot worst.

## Side Effects Valley

### Destruction of the Temple

Well, Satan here we go again back to Nashville and Vanderbilt to see the doctor again. I wonder what he will think now that I have broken loose and attacked his patient's spinal column. I bet he will try to contain me with those nasty chemotherapy drugs. He might as well get ready because I plan to fight that Chemo with all my might. I dread Chemo and steroids, and that's why I smoldered so long. If Miss smarty pants Charlaine had not gotten that massage, I would have allowed her to smolder longer. But when I found that defect in her spine, I just had to spread on over there to that organ. Satan tried to take her voice, so he enticed me to attack her cervix.

I hope he realizes that we just finished seven rounds of radiation. Her doctor told her that if she did not get some treatment soon that she would find herself in a wheelchair. He suggested the radiation to get her through the Thanksgiving and start the chemotherapy after the holidays. I was in favor of delaying all the treatment. I have never been, nor will I ever be, grateful for Chemo. It tries to destroy me, and no matter how hard I fight it, sometimes it wipes me out.

I know Charlaine looked at this smoldering stage of her Myeloma as a blessing because it is the reward for her annual checkup. With regular checkups, cancer and other health problems can be spotted before they become significant issues. When that happens, I hardly have a fighting chance to do much damage or spread to other organs.

Well, let us look back on this cancer path. We smoldered in the valley and headed up the mountain to metastasis where I attacked the spinal column. Now, we are facing the ugly side effects from that strong dose of chemo.

I heard Charlaine tell her nephew that she was troubled about taking the Chemo because her spirit was uneasy. The package itself gave her negative vibes when the postman delivered it. She said she felt an electric impulse when he placed the package in her hand. She signed for it and immediately put it on the altar in her prayer closet.

I thought I would hold off on further destruction. She was still waiting on that miraculous cure, so I will be patient and wait with her. Anything is better than those Chemo infusions. When the cure does not happen, she will have to depend on the Chemo. You know that I would be happy if she chose not to treat herself and continued to wait on that spiritual cure. Chemo only cramps my style and makes me weak. It keeps me from reaching her organs. Her doctor will try to kill me!

> I wonder why He did not stop me or heal her Himself. If He loves her so much, why did he allow me to continue in her body all this time?

In a conversation with her husband, she told him she was afraid of all the warnings about the Chemo. She decided to quench her fears by meditating more and walking with God. It was during her quiet time in Montego Bay that she realized that it was God who had brought her through this valley. It was there in Montego Bay that she wondered why God had not healed her miraculously of cancer. She would get out on the beach each day with her healing scriptures and the Bible to read, study, and meditate on His word.

I heard her questioning God as she began to search to see if there were flaws that were preventing Him from responding to her prayer for healing. She reminded herself each day of her support scripture to let God be in control of her life to and make sure that she was not operating out of selfish pride or control. She soon realized, to walk with God, she had to let Him lead because he knows her future. OK, that means He must have known my plans to attack as well.

I wonder why He did not stop me or heal her Himself. If He loves her so much, why did he allow me to continue in her body all this time? Hey, I am Cancer, what the heck do I care why He did not heal her. Whether He heals her or not, this planned Chemo treatment is going to be devastating for me. I got smart and decided not to attack to give her more time to pray for a healing because God's healing means I simply go away with the Chemo. I think that will be best for the both of us.

I held all attacks and watched her while she waited and prayed, prayed and waited until the pain became unbearable. She started the chemotherapy on November thirtieth and the first week went just great. No side effects so far and she bragged as to how well she was doing. MM was handling the treatments too, but I was no match for the Chemo. I was downright uncomfortable every time I had to put up with those infusions. I became weaker and weaker with each treatment.

It looks like she bragged on her chemo treatment too soon because the next week, she began to see the side effects of the Chemo. Her lips began to blister with little white bumps, and I heard her tell her daughter that her throat was getting sore. Her daughter suggested that she go to the emergency room but, she did not want to go. It was late Friday evening, and she did not want to disrupt the family plans for the weekend. You know how long they take at the ER!

She decided (instead of listening to her daughter, she took control) to call the pharmacy who distributed the Chemo to inform them of her condition and ask for help. I heard them tell her to purchase this medicated cream from the drug store and apply it to her lips as needed. The next morning, I saw her looking at her lips in the mirror to see if the cream had helped her swollen lips. Her lips were not painful, but she noticed that her throat was sore and the blisters had spread to the inside of her mouth. She could hardly swallow so she had her daughter call her niece, Mona a pharmacist and she prescribed her an oral rinse for her throat. She purchased the rinse and began to use it immediately with the hope of being able to eat without pain. The medicine she prescribed numbed her throat, and she could not feel the

pain of swallowing as she tried to enjoy her weekend.

This was the same medication her radiation
doctor prescribed after treating her cervix. I remember the doctor telling her that he had six
rounds of Chemo scheduled and there would be
three infusions per month in each round. I thought
to myself again, they are trying to kill me. That
much Chemo might wipe me completely out, and I
do not have eternal life in the Kingdom. In fact, I
am told there will be no disease or sickness there.

I kept waiting all weekend for something
sweet but, she barely ate her dinner. I needed that
sugar for energy. I was weak and uncomfortable
too. I could see the side effects in the mirror, and
I did not know how many more of those Chemo
infusions I could take. I became self-centered and
not Charlaine-centered.

One thing I noticed about Charlaine is her
love of family. She refused to interrupt the weekend with a visit to the emergency room. Weak as
I was, she got me out of bed early Monday morning though preparing to go to the ER. It was rain-
ing and dreary outside. You could see the light-
ning behind the clouds before the daylight ap-
peared. Charlaine had no respect for the fact that
this was the perfect morning for us to sleep in because she had waited long enough, if not too long,

to see about the effects of her medications.

She decided to get to the hospital early, so she rode to Vanderbilt with her son-in-law. Charlaine is considerate of family times and obligations. Her son-in-law asked if she would be alright or if she needed him to wait with her in the ER until her daughter came. Even though she was fearful, she told him to go on to work. He dropped her off and went to work knowing that his wife planned on coming to the ER after she got their daughter, Madison off to school.

Her daughter wrestled with the thought of why her mother had not gone to the ER sooner. Satan told her to observe her mother's need to be independent and in control. Satan knew that when she thinks she is in control, that is when he can control her. God allows her to "do her thing" uninterrupted when that is her will. Her mother should have gone to the ER on Friday when she first noticed the blisters on her lips. I am sure her daughter appreciated her not disrupting their weekend, but I could see she was genuinely worried about her mom.

She does not know it yet, but her back is about to show the effects of the radiation. I won't take credit for the rash, just the metastasis. I thought I had done enough damage, but everything wants to be noticed. I have effects, radiation has its effects, and Chemo has its effects. I really could not take the credit for the rash or blisters because none of that was caused by me. I am an organ destroyer myself.

Old MM was very kind and considerate to allow Charlaine five years of smoldering. She got through the Mount Metastasis, but here come those nasty side effects from the Chemo. When she was taking her treatments, she noticed all the radiation patients had some sort of mark on their body. Radiation can cause a rash or clusters of small red bumps on the skin. Well, speaking of rash, there is the mark of a reddish rash rising to the surface of her upper back and breasts.

Well, it has been fun having a voice and letting you see from MM (cancer's) perspective how I metastasized and affected Charlaine's body on her journey. She will continue telling you more about her radiation and Chemo side effects in the next chapter, Emergency Room. Since it was the side effects from the Chemo which hospitalized her, it is best to let her share the story about her hospital stay. She can describe the destruction of "the temple" of her body a lot better than I can. She calls it the temple of the Holy Ghost.

I count it a privilege and honor to have had this opportunity to speak because there are two sides to every story and I am glad you got the chance to hear my side of the journey.

# CHAPTER 8:
# EMERGENCY ROOM

*Yea, though I walk through the Valley of the Shadow of Cancer, I felt fearful and all alone.*

I cried out as they wheeled me into the Emergency Room, "Oh my God! I need you to help me! Where are you, God? Where are you? You promised me, and I am standing on your promises right now Lord, Right now. I feel so alone, Lord help me, help me!"

The doctors and interns could not help but stare at my bloody red lips puffed with puss and inflammation. What they could not see was the red rash scattered across my back. What mainly got their attention was my mouth. As I lay on the bed in the emptiness of the treatment room, I looked back on my journey to see when fear first attacked me. I remembered the day the UPS carrier delivered the package of Chemo. I questioned myself about taking the drug. Once again, I cried out,

> *I am all alone. God, where are you? You told me to take that chemo and look at me! I need you now LORD, where are you? Answer me!!!*

Looking for God changed my selfish focus. When my focus changed, I was comforted by the scripture I received to relieve my fear. I had fought off anger ever since the side effects became visible. I took a deep breath and tried to focus on God's promises and the promise he made about my first fear.

I thought of the scripture that says every-thing belongs to God. I present my body to God for it is the temple of the Living God. "God dwells in me, and His life permeates my spirit, soul, and body so that I am filled with the fullness of God daily." (John 14:20) Even though I did not quite understand the scripture, it brought me comfort.

My thoughts were rapid, and I could feel that I was still not comfortable about my condition. Then I thought of all people, I should be able to calm myself down because that is what I do as a counselor. Our minds are much like the computer when we use our visualization. I mentally pulled up my counseling tools. I recalled the Steps for Relieving Stress and the Art of Relaxation. I be-gan to take deep breaths and focused on my body becoming heavy with each breath starting with the top of my head to the bottom of my feet. By the time I finished this relaxation technique, I was comforted. I was repeating the 23rd Psalm when the doctor entered the room saying, "What have we here?"

The ER doctor asked if I was allergic to any medications and asked if I had taken any new medications. I shared that I had been taking Chemo drugs for Cancer. He immediately told me to stop the Chemo because he was afraid I was either having a side effect from the medication or had developed SJS. Don't you just love the fact that some doctors assume you know medical terminology!

I realized that I was calm and sensible when I asked, "SJS what is that?" He explained that it's better known as "Steven Johnson's Syndrome." I never heard of it. He said that it is a deadly viral infection as he left the room.

Word must have spread throughout the ER that a patient was there with SJS. Several of the medical staff came to the room for some reason or another. One student intern came in the treatment room with his cell phone and asked permission to take a picture of my lips. My first reaction was no, thinking I might see myself on Facebook. I asked the student intern what he knew about SJS and what he planned to do with the picture. He immediately said that they have studied the disease and the seriousness of it, but they did not have a visual of it. He promised not to publish the picture without my written consent if he later needed it for his medical journal. I gave him permission after covering my eyes with a brown paper towel to hide my identity. I asked him how serious is serious. He said SJS results in death.

Speaking of cell phones, I took mine and looked up the SJS disease. I learned that Steven-Johnson Syndrome, also called SJS is a rare but severe condition. Most often, it is a severe reaction to a medicine taken. It causes your skin to blister and peel. It affects your mucous membranes, too. Blisters can also form inside your mouth and body, making it hard to eat, swallow, or even urinate. I could hardly eat, but I had no problem urinating.

The ER doctor told me that getting treated right away would help protect my skin and other organs from lasting damage. He asked if I had had a fever or felt like I had the flu. My response was no. There were visible blisters on my mouth, and they were red and painful. The doctor asked me to stop taking the chemo.

I later learned that the antibiotic drugs they prescribed to protect me from infections were medications that could cause SJS. I discovered that radiation treatments could also cause SJS and I did have seven rounds of radiation before starting my Chemotherapy. None of the doctors or staff had mentioned it as a side effect. One thing I learned from this experience is to question the doctor when you do not understand his medical terms and use your cell phone to look up anything you need to find. It is as simple as googling:

<u>www.whatIneedtoknow.com</u>

## DESTRUCTION OF THE TEMPLE

The Radiation affected my back with rash and the Chemo disfigured my face. My mouth, lips, and skin were affected by the strong doses of chemo. When I looked in the mirror, I looked like a character that could have easily played in a "Monster Movie." I honestly did not look like myself at all. I thought to myself, it is good I am up early and leaving before my grandchildren can see me like this. The drugs destroyed my temple.

I arrived at the Vanderbilt ER and was admitted on a Monday. I will never forget it for it was one of the most frightening ordeals of my life. It was truly an emergency. I arrived with blisters inside my mouth, outside on my lips and a radiation rash on my neck and back. By Tuesday, I realized my temple was destroyed, when my vital signs were failing. I was not in any pain, and I was nodding off to sleep only to be awakened by the nurse or aid taking my blood pressure, temperature, and heart rate. My blood pressure kept dropping.

When I look back to the events that took place in the hospital, I realized that all of this was an enactment of the death and burial of Christ. They destroyed His Temple, and His Father raised Him from the tomb on the third day. That scripture He gave me, John 2:19, became very apparent. It was at this point that I declared the destruction of (my body) the Temple. They rushed me to the Intensive Care Unit late that evening after my blood pressure dropped and they could not get it to rise and stabilize.

**(ICU) INTENSIVE CARE UNIT** — The ICU was representative of my tomb or the grave. I was physically in the world, but spiritually I was dead. Here are the accounts of the events which occurred there. I spent exactly three days in the ICU while being treated for a deadly viral infection known as SJS, Steven Johnson Syndrome. The three days represent the days I spent in the ICU (tomb).

## IN THE ICU TOMB

I was taken to the ICU Tomb late Tuesday night after spending Monday in the Emergency Room before being transported to a regular room. I started having trouble with my blood pressure on Tuesday, and because they were not able to stabilize my pressure, I was transported to the ICU. My temple was completely destroyed (dead). My daughter told me how the Vanderbilt staff worked diligently to revive my vitals. It was almost like when you stop breathing and need CPR. I had to have a blood transfusion, but I had little recollection of Day 1. My daughter helped me recall most of the details.

She shared with me that the nurses and assistants were treating my rash and blisters with a creamed prescribed by the ER doctor. My lips were tender and would bleed when I tried to eat. They were very swollen and had begun to dry up. On Thursday, my lips were drying up, and a scab was starting to form on them. My lips were crusty with a dark red blood covering them.

We begin the countdown with day 1 on Wednesday.

**Wednesday, Day I** — Now, I woke up in the ICU which I considered my tomb. They laid me there on a Wednesday, and I remember thinking God said that He would never leave me or forsake me. Even when I feel alone, He is there because I carry Him in my heart at all times. This is what the devil had me overlook when I arrived at the ER. He wanted me to be afraid because fear weakens your faith. I am an overcomer because, in that emergency room, I overcame the devil, the world, and my flesh.

It was a frightening time, but I remembered the woman with the issue of blood, who just touched the hem of Jesus' garment because she knew if she could just touch Him she would be made whole. She was made whole not from touching Jesus' robe, but because she had faith and knew that if she touched Jesus, she would be healed. In remembrance of that, I stretched both hands to the Lord and surrendered my fear. "Father, I stretch my hands to you, Lord, there is no other help I know and if you withdraw from me whether shall I go"? The hospital staff was working on me, collecting blood samples for the lab. Tests would either rule out or confirm the tentative diagnosis of SJS Steven Johnson Syndrome, the deadly viral infection that takes over your body, resulting in death.

My temple was destroyed, and I was buried in the ICU Tomb until Friday, the third day. The scabs were lifting, and by Friday I was feeling better after getting the blood transfusion.

**Thursday, Day 2** — They asked permission to give me blood on Thursday. I was a little hesitant about the blood transfusion, so I prayed before consulting with my niece, Mona Finley. Mona is a Pharmacist, and she suggested I check on a bloodless solution fluid as an alternative to increase my blood. When the doctor and team of students came to see me on their rounds, I asked about the alternative option mentioned by my niece, and they agreed it would be appropriate, but the procedure did not yield immediate results. The doctor explained that people who have severe bone marrow disease may not be responsive because they don't have enough blood-producing cells in their bone marrow so the transfusion would be a better choice. He said that as a Myeloma patient, I could expect frequent needs for blood and that I might as well get used to blood transfusions. I remembered my grandmother always saying, "I am an overcomer by the Blood of the Lamb and the word of my testimony." I told the doctor I would like to pray about the transfusion.

Before noon, the doctor returned to see if I agreed to the blood transfusion and I gave him the "go ahead." They came and drew more blood to match my blood, but I remember wondering why they are still drawing my blood because I am O positive so matching my blood should be easy and quick. Boy, was I wrong! It was taking so long, I asked the nurse about it, and she checked the chart and saw that it had been ordered. She commented that it should not take longer than a couple of hours because of my blood type, but it took all day. I thought I will not worry or be anxious because God's timing is perfect. Matching the blood took all day, and I was weak, but I stayed calm and knew God was controlling the match. It was on Thursday evening that I began to feel better after my vitals stabilized. My daughter, her husband, and the grandkids came to visit me during the ICU afternoon visitation period.

She brought me an electric blanket because I had complained of being cold. Myeloma patients deal with anemia, and that can cause you to feel cold when everyone else is comfortable. They brought me flowers and the grandkids had made me get-well cards. I was glad to see them, and they were happy to see me. They were full of questions about my illness, and I tried to give answers as elementary as I could. They truly brightened my afternoon. The electric blanket was so comforting; I had no problem resting well after an interrupted night of examinations and monitoring procedures.

**Friday, Day 3** — (the third day) in the Intensive Care Unit (ICU):

Early in the afternoon, I finally got the blood transfusion. My daughter called and said the granddaughters were missing their Gigi. They had made me more cards and wanted to bring them to the hospital. They were always doing things to lift my spirit or brighten my day. I told my daughter that I would probably be moving back to a regular hospital room and asked her to bring my bag with my devotion favorites. I had been using my Bible app on my cell phone but, I asked her to look in my car and bring my Bible.

I prayed, meditated on God's Word and felt the urge to speak over myself, "I believe my immunity is getting stronger day by day. I speak life to my immune system. I forbid confusion in my immune system. The same Spirit that raised Christ from the dead dwells in me and quickens my immune system with the life and wisdom of God, which guards the life and health of my body."

> **CANCER IS NO MATCH FOR GOD BECAUSE HE IS SOVEREIGN**

"Body, I speak the Word of Faith to you. I demand that every organ perform a perfect work, for you are the temple of the Holy Ghost; therefore, I charge you in the name of the LORD Jesus Christ and by the authority of God's holy Word to heal me and make me whole in Jesus' Name." (Proverbs 12:18 Paraphrased)

Vanderbilt is a teaching hospital, so doctors and students make late rounds. When they visited my room that evening, I had just finished the blood transfusion that afternoon. I thought I would be moving back to a hospital room, but God raised me out of the ICU tomb on the third day as He promised. I understood the confusion in my immune system. I realized that the same Spirit that raised Christ from the dead dwells in me and quickened my immune system. That same spirit had guarded the life and the health of my body. He kept the promise to raise me up in three days.

Cancer is no match for God because he is Sovereign. He is Omniscient and knows all things. He is Omnipresent appears everywhere at the same time. He is Omnipotent and can do all things. I adore the LORD for He watched over me for five years in the valley. He was there during Mount Metastasis and protected my organs from crippling damage and here in the Valley of Side Effects He spared me from a deadly viral infection, SJS. He led me safely through the valley of the shadow of death after giving me a grip on fear in the emergency room. I now have a greater respect for the comforting Psalm 23.

Life is so full of unanswered questions. Who gets dismissed on the same day of blood transfusion to go HOME? Who gets discharged to go home from ICU? The nurse could not explain it. When things are unexplainable, they are considered to be "miraculous," and the only other answer is God. God needs no explanation for the miracles that He performs.

**SETBACK** — I say unto you that after four months of Chemo I had to start all over on a new Regimen of Chemotherapy. I had to undergo six more months of Chemo inclusive of fifty-two infusions.

There was no need for crying or worrying because of God's promises and His actions. I often wondered "Why Me Lord?" These setbacks were God's way of saying, "Why not you my child?" It was His way of getting my attention, to let me know that He wanted me to declare His works by sharing my testimony for Healing. Despite the setback, the Spirit revealed how God had favored me to be a showcase of His light and hope of healing.

Each day I spend time alone in prayer, and that's when I can see God in the future, and it looks better, so much better. Therefore, I witness and give this testimony of the fact that God keeps his promises, performs miracles and He is still in the healing business.

I cried out to the LORD when I needed Him and "He showed up and showed out" and proved that His promises are true. And if the Spirit of Him who raised Jesus from the dead is living in us, He who raised Christ from the dead will also give life to our mortal bodies because of His Spirit living in us. (Romans 8:11)

He molded me in His own image and taught me that He was in me and me in Him. The same Spirit that raised Christ from the dead dwells in me. He raised me from ICU to Home on the third day.

# CHAPTER 9:
# KNOW GOD'S PURPOSE

*In search of the purpose for my trial.*

Remembering how God has forgiven all my iniquities; He has healed me from a deadly viral infection; He has redeemed my life from destruction; He has transformed me with the blood of the Lamb and healed my body.

I believe that there is a purpose for everything in life. In search of my purpose, I had to know who I am. I had to know God and have a relationship with Him. I established that relationship by reading His Word. It is important for those with chronic illnesses to develop a relationship with Him because He gives us Hope. Once I built that relationship with God, I developed a stronger "will to live" and was able to trust Him to lead me through the trials of my journey with cancer.

My cancer diagnosis has a purpose, and I still spend time with God, reading His word and meditating on the scriptures.

> *In my desperation, I pray, the Lord listens and saves me from all my troubles. He frees me from all my fears and leads me to examine the situation in search for a purpose. (Psalm 34:4-6)*

My purpose is generated from my skills and talents learned from life experiences. It is a culmination of all the things I like to do and the people I like doing them with. Have you given any thought to what you love to do? I love explaining things to people, and this love has manifested itself as a teaching gift. I enjoy helping people solve their personal problems that demand Godly communication skills and spiritual logical thinking skills. Hence, part of my life's purpose is to empower people (cancer victims) who are not aligned with Christ to start a relationship with Him, for He is our hope for tomorrow. He tells us to "count it all joy," (James 1:2-4) "Listen my brethren; count it all joy when you fall into various trials, knowing that the testing of your faith produces patience. But let patience have its perfect work, that you may be perfect and complete, lacking nothing (when we experience our cancer journey or have other trials or chronic diseases)."

I meditated on the scriptures day and night and night and day until the Holy Spirit answered me with Psalm 118:17, "You will not die but live to declare the Works of the LORD." This scripture gave me comfort. I knew God had a purpose for my battle with cancer and I was willing to accept it as a learning experience as His purpose for my life. Now I am committed to serving His Purpose.

When life gets hard, we tend to get upset and wonder how soon the difficulty will end. But God wants us to focus on Him in times of trouble. It is best to be God-Centered and not self-Centered. As we focus on God, we will discover that He is doing important spiritual work during these "storms." I knew that I would be pruned, sifted, and shaped for His purpose and was willing to accept the challenge.

Life is a series of problems or trials. Either you are in one now, are just coming out of one, or are getting ready to go into another one. The reason for this is that God is interested in building our character. I am a believer that problems or trails help build Godly character and draw us closer to God. God is more interested in making our life holy than He is in making our life happy. We can be reasonably happy here on earth, but that is not the goal of life. The goal of life is to grow in character, in Christ-likeness. You may ask, what is Christ-likeness? It is having and displaying the character of Jesus Christ. All Christians are commanded to worship the Lord, care for one another, and share in the work of spreading the gospel. God's followers are also given spiritual gifts to use in building up other believers or those struggling with trials of life

These truths are the basis for my view of life. I find myself growing in the grace and knowledge of Jesus Christ. Forgiving others has become a possibility—and dying of self a more common occurrence. Ungodly traits have faded away and been replaced by the fruit of the Spirit. I find that

His character is defined in Galatians 5:22-23. I display them each day on my breastplate as a remnant of the armor of the Holy Spirit.

Because I have built a strong relationship with Christ, the Holy Spirit produces the fruit of God's spirit in me. The fruits of goodness, joy, kindness, LOVE, meekness, peace, patience, self-control, and temperance are all characteristics of Jesus Christ. These characteristics are necessary for discipline on my journey with cancer. The greatest of these characteristics is LOVE. God's love speaks for itself. It shows how much we can trust him.

Ellen G. White, says it best in **Our Father Cares**, p.27 *Love for Others*

"Be ye, therefore, followers of God, as dear children; and walk in love, as Christ also hath loved us, and hath given himself for us an offering and a sacrifice to God for a sweet-smelling savor. Ephesians 5:1-2. You are to trust God as dear children, to be obedient to all His requirements, walking in love as Christ also hath loved us. Love was the element in which Christ moved and walked and worked. He came to embrace the world in the arms of His love. We are to follow the example set by Christ, and make Him our pattern until we shall have the love for others as He has manifested for us. He seeks to impress us with this profound lesson of love. If your hearts have been given to selfishness, let Christ imbue you with His love. He desires that we shall trust and love Him fully, and encourages, yes, even commands, that we shall love others as He has given us an example. He has made love the badge of our discipleship. This is the measurement to which you are to reach, "Love one another; as I have loved you." What height, what depth and breadth of love! This love is not merely to embrace a few favorites; it is to reach to the lowliest and humblest of God's creatures. I know we must love especially those who are battling cancer and other diseases."

Wait on the LORD! It is not easy waiting on the LORD, and for that reason, I adopted as my daily devotional scripture Proverbs 3:5-6, *Trust in the LORD with all my heart and lean not on my own understanding but in all my ways acknowledge Him to direct my path.* It is this verse of scripture that keeps me grounded. One of the first things I had to do in search of God's purpose for my life was to examine myself. In the examination, two conditions were unaligned with God. These were the conditions of Control and

Pride. Neither of these conditions is favorable or any part of the "fruits of the spirit" which represents the characteristics of Jesus Christ. I conditioned these behaviors with much prayer and bathing my mind and thoughts with quotes of Positive Attitude:

*Keep your thoughts Positive*
*because your thoughts become your*
*Words,*
*your words become your Behavior*
*your Behavior become your Habits*
*your Habits become your Values*
*your Values become your Destiny*
*- Mahatma Gandhi*

*So much in life depends on our attitude the way we choose to see things and respond to others makes all the difference.*
*-President Thomas A. Manson*

My battle with Cancer has led me to believe that God has chosen me to live in such a time as this. I must give my best to Him. I will magnify and praise the Lord, and He will use me to showcase His Love, grace, and mercy to educate, encourage and empower others. I hope to tenaciously declare the Works of the Lord and be obedient to His will.

The Holy Spirit guided me to the truth. The

days in the wilderness provided me comfort because the Holy Spirit nourished my soul. I was
like that of a baby hungry for milk (the Word). He,
the Holy Spirit led me to this Psalm:

*Have mercy upon me, O God, according
to Thy loving-kindness: According unto
the multitude of Thy tender mercies blot
out my transgressions... For I know my
transgressions: and my sin is ever before
me...Purge me with hyssop, and I shall
be clean: wash me, and I shall be whiter
than snow... Create in me a clean heart,
O God; and renew a right spirit within
me. Cast me not away from Thy
presence, and take not Thy Holy Spirit
from me. Restore unto me the joy of Thy
salvation, and uphold me with Thy free
spirit... Deliver me from bloodguiltiness,
O God, Thou God of my salvation: And
my tongue shall sing aloud of Thy
righteousness. (Psalm 51:1-14)*

I kept thinking of the scripture the Holy
Spirit revealed at the MEET Ministry Home. This
is the place I chose to prepare me for my change
of life. I accepted their goal for me. Their goal was
to open all channels of elimination of waste from
my bowels, kidney, lungs, blood, liver, and lymph.

The program provided nutritional support including instruction on how to plant and grow a vegetable garden to avoid pesticides and toxins. This is the place where He again revealed this scripture (Psalm 118:17) You will not die but live to declare the works of the LORD. I feel like the spirit of the LORD is upon me, because he anointed me to declare his works to the world. The Holy Spirit is at work all the time, and I am so glad I learned how to be filled with God's spirit and how to pray for healing.

While getting treatments at Vanderbilt Hospital, I met a man who was so distraught from the devastating news that he was dying of cancer and had discussed Hospice Care with his doctor. We were at the check-in desk, and I was prompted by the Holy Spirit to pray for him. We moved out into the hallway, and the registration clerk asked if she could join her husband and me. We gathered around in a circle holding hands and before I prayed declaring the Works of God and his healing power. I asked the man if he believed that Christ died on the cross for His sins so that he could have eternal life in the Kingdom of God. After he had responded that he did believe, I prayed for him.

I gave them one of the million-dollar-bill

tracts that I distribute throughout the hospital during my visits to the infusion lab with the plan for salvation on the bill's backside and a million dollars on its front. It truly gets their attention. It's a great way to introduce Christ. I told her how important it is that her husband gets plenty of sunlight and how his organs will thirst for water. She responded that she was trying to get him to drink more water.

I encouraged his wife to pray for her husband every morning. I believed prayer would focus them on God for the day. I came across their path a few months later and smiled at him and said, you look much better. His wife stated that they were praying and believing God. I spoke a couple of healing scriptures over him and applauded their positive attitude. We exchanged cell phone numbers, and I told his wife that I would text her some healing scriptures.

I felt the Holy Spirit using me on clinic days at Vanderbilt Hospital in Nashville to proclaim God's goodness as a means of declaring His works. I feel as though He set me free and protected me from the infusion sickness so I could proclaim His wonderful works to those cancer victims in the clinic. Many of them ask me if I have cancer and I respond, "I have God" and what they saw in me was His favor because of my belief. I am empowered by the spirit to continue a conversation with them. Everyone who sees me for the first time admires the fact that I do not look or act like I have cancer. My response to them is always, "I Love Jesus" and He anoints me to showcase His Love. I learned that this is what God meant when He said I was to declare His Works.

One day I received a call from the young man whom I had prayed for at the Vanderbilt Cancer Infusion Clinic. He called to tell me he was feeling better and his doctor had seen a slight improvement. I gave a shout, "Praise the Lord!" He thanked me, and I told him all the thanks and glory is to God who is our Healer. I keep tabs on him through the registration clerk and an occasional cell phone call. He is still living and only gets the infusion once a month as I do. We both acknowledged how God answers prayer. I want to be obedient to God and tell others about His healing powers. I must fight the devil off as I proclaim that I am an overcomer by the blood of the Lamb. With God's help, I ask the Holy Spirit to help me overcome the world, the flesh, and the devil. This cancer battle is not mine, it is the LORD's. I trust God for He is my healer. No matter what my body is telling me, I trust God to heal me and fill me with overwhelming joy.

*Jesus is the Lord of my life. Sickness and*

*disease have no power over me. I am*
*forgiven and free from SIN and GUILT. I*
*am dead to sin and alive unto righteous-*
*ness. (Col. 1:21-22)*

I no longer need to search for His Purpose for my Life, for now, I know that He made me on purpose, for His purpose of (PCO) Providing Christ-Centered Options to His people who are struggling with their trials of life. This testimony of my trial should provide evidence of God's power to heal while respecting His Will.

PCO Counseling Service was established more than 25 years ago and continues to be the avenue God has chosen as Purpose for me to minister to the people. He taught me Christ-like character necessary for counseling people "God's Way." This trial is His way of showcasing His Love, Grace, and Mercy so that others can see that the same Spirit that raised Him from the dead abides in me, as I abide in Him.

*"My people perish for lack of knowledge."*
*(Hosea 4:6)*

It is clear now that God has anointed me to share my trial to educate His children about cancer. I am to encourage those who are going through to trust God and put their faith in Him to fight their battle and empower them to wait on the LORD.

He will never leave us or forsake us. Even though we have gained knowledge, it is OK to question cancer, but be encouraged to meditate daily, journal your thoughts as you serve God's purpose for your life, and be empowered to tell His story.

When I look back over my life, I see how God has smiled on me. I could have been dead and buried in my grave, but he chose to shape me and mold me for His Purpose. I will be forever grateful for His Love and favor over my life.

# CHAPTER 10:
# NUTRITION, HEALTH, AND WELLNESS

*God's plan of biblical foods*

Because I have his promises, I will cleanse my body of everything that can defile my body or spirit. And let us work toward complete holiness because we fear God just as it says in 2 Corinthians 7:1.

I learned many things at the MEET Ministry Camp. I learned that God truly cares how I treat my body and He has given me a free health plan to go by in the Bible. When I obey God's Biblical Plan for nutrition, health, and wellness I can have abundant health and longer life. This is what all cancer victims seek and strive to achieve.

The Bible rates health right near the top of the list in importance. A person's mind, spiritual nature, and body are all interrelated and interdependent. What affects one affects others. If the body is misused, the mind and spiritual nature cannot become what God planned they should be, and you will not be able to live an abundant life. (John 10:10), the thief's purpose is to steal

> IGNORING GOD'S "OPERATIONS MANUAL" CAN RESULT IN DISEASE, TWISTED THINKING, AND BURNED-OUT STRESSED LIVES...

and kill and destroy. My purpose is to give them a rich and satisfying life.

God gave us health principles for a reason. *"The LORD commanded us to observe all these statutes, to fear the LORD our God, for our good always, that He might preserve us alive." (Deuteronomy 6:24)* We find this wisdom in *Exodus 23:25. "You shall serve the LORD your God, and He will bless your bread and your water. And I will take sickness away from the midst of you"* God gave health principles because He knows what is best for our human body (His temple).

The automobile manufacturer places an operation manual in the glove compartment of each new car because they know what is best for their creation. Well, God created us and don't you think He knows what is best for us? Guess what our operation manual is? It is the Bible. Ignoring God's "operations manual" can result in disease, twisted thinking, and burned-out stressed lives, just as abusing a car can lead to serious car trouble. I have learned that we can save our health by following God's principles. God gives us free will, and if we choose to cooperate, God can use these great health laws to significantly reduce and eliminate the effects of the diseases of Satan. (Psalm 103:2-3) Let all that I am praise the LORD; may I never forget the good things he does for me. He forgives all my sins and heals all my diseases.

Once we take on God's Plan and follow the instruction manual, we will eat and drink differently. We will choose only "what is good." If the Bible says a thing is not fit to eat, it's God's Word for a good reason. He is our loving Father and not a dictator. All His counsel is for our good always. The Bible promises God will not withhold any good thing from us who walk uprightly. If God withholds a thing from us, it is because it is not good for us. I learned this principle best from my experience in Jamaica with the discounted massage. God was withholding the coupon because He knew that massage would not be good for me. When I ignored Him, Satan took me up the Mountain to Metastasis and down the Valley of Side Effects. I know the importance of obeying God when he withholds, it is because He knows what is best for me.

The subject of healing appears in scripture throughout the whole Bible, from Genesis to Revelation. If we are wise, we will become acquainted with God's Plan and heed His instructions. Each letter in "God's Plans" leads us to a scripture verse in the Bible that details the importance of the plan. Some say that the BIBLE is our **B**asic **I**nstructions **B**efore **L**eaving **E**arth.

*Lord, You have blessed my food and water and have taken sickness away from me. Therefore I will fulfill the number of my days in health. (Exodus 23:25, 26)*

His plan is outlined in the Bible in the following scriptures (paraphrased): G O D' S P L A N

## G - Godly Trust    Genesis 2:17

*Except for the tree of Knowledge, of good and evil, if you eat its fruit, you are sure to die.*

## O - Open Air    Genesis 1:6-7

*And God said, "Let there be a space between the waters, to separate the waters of the heavens from the waters of the earth." And that is what happened. God made this space to separate the waters of the earth from the waters of heaven.*

## D - Daily Exercise    Genesis 2:15

*The LORD God placed the man in the Garden of Eden to work it and take care of it.*

## S - Sunshine    Genesis 1:16

*God made two great lights—the greater light to govern the day, and the lesser light to govern the night. He also made the stars.*

## P - Proper Rest    Genesis 2:3

*Then God blessed the seventh day and*

*declared it holy because on it He rested from all the work of creating that he had done.*

## L - **Lots of Water**    Genesis 2:10

*A river watering the garden flowed from Eden, from there it was separated into four Headwaters (branches).*

## A - **Always Temperate**   Genesis 2:16, 17

*And the LORD God commanded the man, 'You are free to eat from any tree in the garden – but you must not eat the tree of the knowledge of good and evil, for when you eat from it, you will certainly die.*

## N - **Nutrition**    Genesis 1:29

*Then God said, "I have given you every seed-bearing plant on the far of the whole earth and every tree that has fruit with seed in it. They will be yours for food.*

The diet God gave people, in the beginning, was fruit, grains, and nuts. Vegetables were added a little later as indicated in Genesis 3:18. "God said, "See I have given of every herb that yields seed of every tree whose fruit yields seeds. Of every tree of the garden, you may freely eat."

Rev. Percy McCray Jr., the Director of Faith-

Based Programs at CTCA, Cancer Treatment Centers of America, has spent more than twenty years ministering to cancer patients and their caregivers. He has identified the foods in the Bible that are rich in natural nourishment for our body.

**Dr. McCray makes no claim these foods will cure cancer.** He says that the foods of biblical times were all natural, unprocessed, fresh foods. In that time, there were no preservatives, pesticides, hormones or antibiotics added to food. For a more complete listing of Rev. Percy McCray's *Biblical Foods* or to get a free download of his book, follow this link: www.HealthHopeandInspiration.

Our fast food culture makes it easy to eat those things that are delicious but not always healthy. It makes dinner and food preparation a thing of the past. Stop being slothful and select fresh food items at the grocery stores. Eating healthy is a planned activity. Consider carefully what food goes into your grocery basket. Now that you know better, you can make better food selections, change your diet, and take a hard look at your lifestyle in general.

# CHAPTER 11:
# LIFESTYLE CHANGES FOR RESTORATION

*Employ the Biblical Health Principles for improved health, better nutrition and achieve wellness.*

Here are twelve biblical health principles that helped me change my lifestyle.

1. Started eating my meals at regular intervals, and do not use animal fat or blood. "Feast (eat) at the proper time." (Ecclesiastes 10:17) "This shall be a perpetual statute; you shall eat neither fat nor blood." (Leviticus 3:17) Fats results in high cholesterol levels and heart attacks.

2. Stopped the habit of overeating. "Put a knife to your throat if you are a man given to appetite." (Proverbs 23:2) Christ specifically warned against "carousing" (intemperance) in the last days. Overeating is a form of intemperance.

3. Learned not to harbor envy or hold grudges. These sinful feelings disrupt body processes. The Bible says that envy is "rottenness to the bones." (Proverbs 14:30) Christ commanded us to clear up grudges that others might hold against us. (Matthew 5:23,24)

4. Maintain a cheerful disposition. "A merry heart does good, like medicine." (Proverbs 17:22) Many diseases from which people suffer are a result of depression. Many cancer victims suffer depression. A cheerful, happy disposition imparts health and prolongs life. I think a positive attitude helps ward off depression as well.

**5.** Put my full trust in the Lord. "Fear of the LORD leads to life." (Proverbs 19:23) Trust in the Lord strengthens health and life. "My son, give attention to my words for they are life to those who find them, and health to all their flesh." (Proverbs 4:20, 22) When we put our trust in God and are Obedient to His commands, we promote good health.

**6.** Learned to balance work and exercise with sleep and rest. "Six days I labor and do all my work, but the seventh day is the Sabbath of the LORD our God." (Genesis 3:19) I don't do any work. It is vain for me to rise early, to sit up late. I was taught to go to bed at 9 p.m. and rise at 6 a.m. at the MEET Ministry health and nutrition camp.

**7.** Keep my body clean because I have His promises. I cleanse my body of everything that can defile it. Isaiah 52:11 commands that I "be clean."

**8.** Am mindful and temperate in all things. I try to be moderate in the use of things that are good. Habits that injure my health break the command "I shall not kill." (1 Corinthians 9:25)

**9.** Avoid things that are harmful to my body, I try to avoid it (1 Corinthians 3:16, 17). I discovered that tea, coffee, and soft drinks that contain the drug caffeine are harmful to my body. Soft drinks are popular because of caffeine and sugar, not the flavor. Many people are sick because of their addiction to coffee, tea, and soft drinks.

**10.** Make mealtime a happy time so that my food will digest properly. The Bible says, "Every man should eat and drink and enjoy the good of all his labor." (Ecclesiastes 3:13) It is the gift of God. Meals with family while sharing conversation, help us to eat slower and enjoy our food.

**11.** Try to be His servant and help those who are in need. When I help the poor and needy, I improve my own health. (Isaiah 58:6-8) When I share my food with the hungry and clothe the naked, my healing improves.

**12.** Strive for healthy living. That is a part of the Bible, and I must strive to change my lifestyle to follow God's health principles to achieve wellness.

*We all sin and come short of the Kingdom of God. I am not perfect in any way. My flesh is weak, but God is mighty, and I choose to let Him lead me. I am striving each day to change my life so that God can use me for His purpose.*

# EPILOGUE:
# WHAT CANCER DID NOT DO

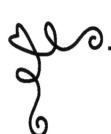

## What Cancer Cannot Do

*Cancer is so limited,*

*It cannot cripple **LOVE***

*It cannot shatter **HOPE***

*It cannot corrode **FAITH***

*It cannot eat away **PEACE***

*It cannot destroy **CONFIDENCE***

*It cannot kill **FRIENDSHIP***

*It cannot shut out **MEMORIES***

*It cannot silence **COURAGE***

*It cannot reduce **ETERNAL LIFE***

*It cannot quench the **SPIRIT***

Author Unknown

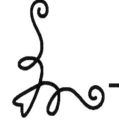
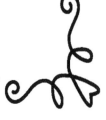

# What Cancer Did Not Do
*Charlaine F. Price*

## Cancer did not cripple my LOVE
*Love is a commandment. We are to love God and our neighbor as ourselves.*

## Cancer did not shatter my HOPE
*Hope is what I have for trusting in God to give me the strength to bear my trials.*

## Cancer did not corrode my FAITH
*Faith is what I needed to trust in God as my Healer.*

## CANCER did not eat away PEACE
*Peace is what God gave me when I went to Him in prayer.*

## Cancer did not destroy CONFIDENCE
*Confidence is what I have when I study God's Word, meditate on his Healing Scriptures and apply His Healing Principles to my life.*

## Cancer did not kill FRIENDSHIP
*Friendship became more valuable than ever before when I realized the impact of prayer and realized that friends are my Prayer Warriors.*

## Cancer did not shut out MEMORIES
*Memories good and bad will always be cherished because it is the memories of my journey with cancer that have allowed me to provide this declaration of God's Love and protection.*

## Cancer did not silence COURAGE
*Courage is what I develop when all seems lost, and I must press on toward the mark of endurance.*

## Cancer did not reduce ETERNAL LIFE
*Eternal Life is my reward for believing that Christ died for me. I strive to live a God-centered life because I have been saved by the blood of the Lamb, Jesus Christ.*

## Cancer did not quench the SPIRIT
*Spirit is what I pray to be filled with every morning so that I can be in Christ and He can be in me. I know that the same Spirit that raised Christ from the dead dwells in me and raised me from destruction on the third day.*

# Share the Message

If you enjoyed this book, please visit *He Restored My Soul: In the Valley of the Shadow of Cancer* on Amazon.com and leave a review.

Books may be purchased through the website www.charlaineprice.com

If you would like to see a pictorial history of Charlaine's journey through the Valley of Cancer, go to www.charlaineprice.com.

Proceeds will be used to provide space and materials for weekly Cancer Support Groups.

Speaking engagements may be requested via email: **pcocounseling@comcast.net** or mail:

PCO COUNSELING SERVICE
Heritage V Building
5916 Brainerd Road, Suite 110
Chattanooga, Tennessee 37411

# WORKS CITED

Capps, Charles, God's Creative Power for Healing, Charles Capps Ministries, England, Arkansas

Gruenwald, Bobby, creator "You Version," Bible App. 2007

McCray Jr., Rev. Percy, Director of Faith-Based Programs at CTCA, Cancer Treatment Centers of America. "Foods of the Bible" Podcast Link, HealthHopeandInspriation.com, 2017.

MEET—Missionary Education & Evangelistic Training, Home Life Saving Retreat in Huntington, Tennessee. (MEET Study Notes-" GOD'S PLAN") September 2015.

Price, Charlaine F. "All Cancers Matter" presentation at the American Breast Cancer Awareness Week, Mary Locher Foundation, Chattanooga, State Technical Community College, Chattanooga, Tennessee. (October 2016)

Stanley, Dr. Charles, Pastor In Touch Ministry, New King James Version, "The Charles F. Stanley Life Principles Bible", Thomas Nelson Inc., 1982 Atlanta, GA (In Touch study notes, "Daily Devotion" )2011-2016

Walter, John, President and CEO of the Leukemia & Lymphoma Society (LLS) "Myeloma" publication, White Plains, NY revised 2013

WEB MD, "American Cancer Society's, Most Recent Facts and Figures," (2017 annual report )

Ellen G. White, Prolific Author, Estate" Daily Devotional- "Our Father Cares," p.27 "Love for Others" (MEET Study Notes) September 2015

# INDEX

CPSIA information can be obtained
at www.ICGtesting.com
Printed in the USA
BVHW01s1928050318
509750BV00011B/388/P